THE
REMARKABLE
SURGICAL PRACTICE
OF
JOHN BENJAMIN MURPHY

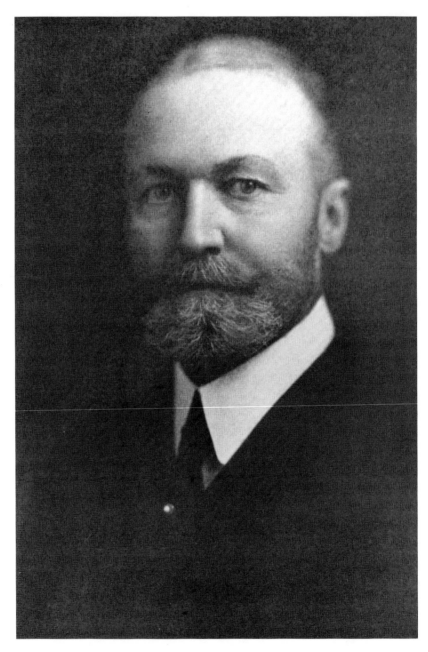

John Benjamin Murphy, M.D., F.A.C.S., F.R.C.S. (Eng.), L.L.D.

THE
REMARKABLE
SURGICAL PRACTICE
OF
JOHN BENJAMIN MURPHY

EDITED BY
Robert L. Schmitz and Timothy T. Oh

UNIVERSITY OF ILLINOIS PRESS
Urbana and Chicago

Publication of this book was made possible in part by the
generous support of Mercy Hospital and Medical Center, Chicago,
especially Sister Sheila Lyne and Mr. Winkle Lee.

This book is printed on acid-free paper.

Library of Congress Cataloging-in-Publication Data

The Remarkable surgical practice of John Benjamin Murphy / edited by
   Robert L. Schmitz and Timothy T. Oh.
      p.   cm.
   Includes bibliographical references.
   ISBN 0-252-01958-X (cl. : alk. paper)
      1. Murphy, JH. B. (John Benjamin), 1857-1916. Surgeons—United
   States—Biography. 3. Surgery—United States—History. 4. Surgery—
   bibliography.
   [DNLM: 1. Murphy, J. B. (John Benjamin), 1857-1916. 2. Surgery—
   biography. 3. Surgery, Operative—methods. WZ 100 M9789]
   RD27.35.M87R46   1993
   617'.092—dc20
   [B]
   DNLM/DLC
   for Library of Congress   92-524
                                                                  CIP

CONTENTS

Foreword
Sr. Sheila Lyne and Lloyd M. Nyhus
vii

Preface
Robert L. Schmitz
ix

Reference System
xi

1. MURPHY'S LIFE
Robert L. Schmitz and Timothy T. Oh
1

2. MURPHY'S PRACTICE IN GENERAL
Robert L. Schmitz, Sr. Christeta Boring, and Milorad M. Cupic
22

3. GENERAL SURGERY
William A. Tito, William H. Blair, and Alejandra Perez-Tamayo
37

4. GYNECOLOGY
Robert L. Schmitz
66

5. NEUROSURGERY
Michael J. Jerva and Robert L. Schmitz
73

6. ORTHOPEDICS
Robert L. Schmitz and Gerald F. Loftus
85

7. THORACIC SURGERY
Frank J. Milloy
119

8. UROLOGY
James J. Burden, Eugene T. McEnery, and Robert L. Schmitz
142

9. VASCULAR SURGERY
Michael J. Verta and Robert L. Schmitz
149

10. INFECTIOUS DISEASES
Warren W. Furey and Robert L. Schmitz
155

11. AN APPRAISAL
Robert L. Schmitz
165

APPENDIX A: THE BIBLIOGRAPHY OF JOHN B. MURPHY
Robert L. Schmitz and Timothy T. Oh
167

APPENDIX B: SELECTED REFERENCES TO JOHN B. MURPHY
Robert L. Schmitz
202

NOTES ON THE CONTRIBUTORS
206

FOREWORD

It has been said that in the early years of Mercy Hospital in Chicago, the trials and triumphs of the hospital paralleled those of the city itself. We could also say that the progress and prominence of Mercy Hospital in that early period were launched by the intensive study, pioneering surgery, and inspired teaching of John Benjamin Murphy.

Dr. Murphy's work in the aftermath of the Haymarket Riot, his involvement with the treatment of Theodore Roosevelt following an assassination attempt, his stimulating performances in the surgical amphitheater, his activities at Mercy Hospital, and many other aspects of his career were all colored with drama and even a little arrogance. These facets of his life are well known. However, the present book provides for the first time a compendium of Murphy's surgical practice, his inventions, his writings, and his clinics. Robert Schmitz and Timothy Oh have assembled the story of Murphy's work ethic and all it involved, as mapped out by the surgeon's successors at Mercy Hospital. As this study demonstrates, Murphy's extraordinary contributions cannot be denied.

Murphy had an important role in the founding of the American College of Surgeons, and between 1892 and 1901 he was a professor of clinical surgery at the College of Physicians and Surgeons. This college became the University of Illinois College of Medicine in 1913. In recent years Mercy Hospital has been a part of the Metropolitan Group Hospitals of the College of Medicine's training program in general surgery, and it has been the keystone of this program. All who are associated with these institutions are proud of the Murphy legacy.

John B. Murphy's dedication to medical care and devotion to medical education were also the objectives of the Sisters of Mercy, beginning in 1852, and have been shared by the medical staff of

Mercy Hospital since its founding. Murphy's example, as put forth in this book, makes us all aware of what is possible in health care through technological advances, research discoveries, and compassionate patient care.

Sr. Sheila Lyne, R.S.M.
Lloyd M. Nyhus, M.D.

PREFACE

John Benjamin Murphy was chief of surgery at Mercy Hospital, Chicago, from 1895 to 1916. Through the generosity of his granddaughter, Mrs. Jeanette Hurley-Haywood Reuben, and the American College of Surgeons, the hospital acquired a sizable number of his papers including working drafts, art work, reprints, letters, clippings, notebooks, ledgers, and surgical logs. In addition, we have his patients' office records for the years 1904 to 1916, three boxes of X-ray plates of his patients, and many flip charts of "before-and-after" patient photographs that he used for teaching.

As we reviewed his papers it became evident that Murphy had made substantially more major contributions to surgery than he is usually credited with and that a comprehensive overview of his practice had never been written. It seemed appropriate to us that we should attempt to prepare such an overview, especially since his influence and many of his innovations are still with us today in such areas as physical examination, experimental surgery, appendicitis, intestinal obstruction, bone grafting, joint surgery, and nerve repair, and in the *Surgical Clinics of North America* and the American College of Surgeons.

Throughout our effort we have had the encouragement of Sister Sheila Lyne, administrator of Mercy Hospital and Medical Center, Chicago; Mrs. Jeanette Reuben; and Lloyd M. Nyhus, professor and head emeritus of the Department of Surgery of the College of Medicine of the University of Illinois at Chicago. Special thanks go to Mary Jane English Schmitz for her support at all stages of this project.

We are grateful to W. B. Saunders Company for permitting us to use many illustrations from the *Surgical Clinics of North America;* to *Surgery, Gynecology, and Obstetrics* for the material in Chapter 7, most of which appeared in volume 171 (November 1990) of that journal; and to the Institute of Medicine of Chicago for granting us permission to use the material in Appendix A that was previously published in its *Proceedings* (volume 42, no. 1, 1989).

Robert L. Schmitz, M.D.
Timothy T. Oh

REFERENCE SYSTEM

In the following chapters, references will be identified according to this system:

1. To the indexed literature: (1) or (1, p. 222).
2. To Murphy's journal articles: JBM plus the number given to the article in Appendix A, e.g., (JBM 25) or (JBM 25, p. 15).
3. To *Surgical Clinics* entries: *SC* plus the number given to the entry in Appendix A, e.g., (*SC* 136) or (*SC* 136, p. 456).
   Abbreviated journal titles used throughout this book are:
   Ann. Surg. = *Annals of Surgery*
   JAMA = *Journal of the American Medical Association*
   Surg. Clin. North Am. = *Surgical Clinics of North America*
   Surg. Gynecol. Obstet. = *Surgery, Gynecology and Obstetrics*

THE
REMARKABLE
SURGICAL PRACTICE
OF
JOHN BENJAMIN MURPHY

1

MURPHY'S LIFE

Robert L. Schmitz and Timothy T. Oh

He was born on December 21, 1857, in a log cabin on a farm near Appleton, Wisconsin, the fifth child of six born to Irish immigrants. His family's financial circumstances were humble at best. He was baptized simply John Murphy.

Life on the farm was rigorous, and young John was expected to do his share. His mother was a staunch Catholic who emphasized morality and discouraged drinking and smoking. This stern beginning conditioned him well for the dedicated, industrious life he was to lead.

To gain his elementary education, John walked eight miles round trip between home and a one-room school each day. After completing grammar school he attended high school in Appleton and worked part time in a drugstore to earn a little money. It was evident quite early that he had a driving urge for knowledge and a stoical ability to work to obtain it. There was never any room for frivolity in his life.

One of his high school teachers, R. H. Schmidt, recognized his talent and hoped to guide him into teaching as a career. But Dr. H. W. Reilly had offices just above the drugstore, and he often called Murphy to assist him in the office and to ride along on house calls. Thus Murphy was introduced to the medical profession, and soon the lad was torn between these two paths.

Following graduation from high school in 1876, Murphy did try a short period as a teacher, but his interest in medicine soon took over and he approached Dr. Reilly to become his preceptor. Reilly was happy to oblige; his fee was two hundred dollars. Murphy had saved some money but had to ask his mother for extra help. In addition to having young Murphy assist him in his office and on his calls, Reilly had him read Gray's *Anatomy* and Draper's *Physiology*. It was a beginning.

A year later, with further moral support and financial help from his mother, Murphy decided to apply to medical school. Besides those in Philadelphia and New York, he considered two in Chicago: Rush Medical College and Chicago Medical College. After much deliberation, he chose to stay near home and applied to Rush, which had received a charter in 1837 and had opened in 1843. Schooling there consisted of a set of lectures which was repeated the second year. Murphy was graduated in 1879 at the age of twenty-two.

As he was nearing adulthood, the lack of a middle name bothered him and he asked several relatives for suggestions. A cousin, Margaret Grimes, suggested Benjamin; the name appealed to him and he added it to his own. As he tried various forms of his new name in his signature, he gradually settled on J. B. Murphy, and so he has been most commonly called since. To his intimates, however, he was plain "J. B."

It was during his medical school years that Murphy grew the full beard that became his trademark. In the beginning it was blond-red in color but as he aged it became a dark gray; he kept it neatly trimmed at all times and carefully parted it in the middle.

The many contentions he had with his colleagues all during his life also began during these years. Arey (1) tells us "he was unpopular as a medical student, his monopolizing of class time by question and argument being interpreted as pure 'show-off.'"

Although further medical training was not required, Murphy appreciated its value and took the oral examination for the very competitive internship at Cook County Hospital, winning first place. While interning, he came to the attention of Dr. Edward W. Lee, who recognized his potential and offered him a partnership at the end of his training period. Murphy joined him in 1881; the population of Chicago at this time was 850,000.

Early in his practice with Dr. Lee, Murphy decided on surgery as a specialty. As soon as Murphy made this choice, Christian Fenger, who had been impressed with him at County Hospital, urged him to study in Europe. With further financial help from his mother, Murphy took off for a *Wanderjahr* in which he was to study at Vienna, Berlin, and Heidelberg with such giants as Theodor Billroth, Carl Schroeder, and Julius Arnold. For six months before he left, Murphy had studied German to prepare himself for his journey. Lee assured him that his job would still be open when he returned.

It was while he was in Vienna that Murphy had a bout of painless hematuria. The professors there diagnosed it as tuberculosis and he prepared to return home. But when the ailment did not recur, he canceled his return and continued on to Berlin instead, later traveling on to Heidelberg. After eighteen months abroad, he finally felt he was ready for a surgical career and sailed for America.

On his homecoming in 1884, he returned to his partnership with Edward Lee and continued with him for several years. One day when Dr. Lee could not make a house call he sent Murphy instead, and that was how J. B. met his future wife, Jeanette "Nettie" Plamondon, the daughter of an affluent industrialist. She was seriously ill with typhoid fever and Murphy attended her diligently until she recovered. By that time they were in love, and they married on November 25, 1885, when she was just eighteen and he was twenty-eight.

His marriage was undoubtedly one of the most significant events in Murphy's early life. Besides bringing him happiness, it lifted him out of his humble financial state and brought him into immediate social prominence. As a wedding present Mrs. Murphy's parents gave the couple a home next door to theirs on fashionable Throop Street. It is often said that Nettie, so proud of her husband, used her connections to engineer much of the publicity Murphy received in the press during his career.

The Murphys' first child, Harold (b. 1886), died in infancy from diphtheria in spite of a tracheostomy. That year, 1887, was a bad one for Murphy because he also lost a sister and two brothers to tuberculosis. Eventually, however, J. B. and Nettie had four lovely daughters, Jeanette (b. 1889, who lived just four years), Cecile (b. 1890), Mildred (b. 1892), and Celeste (b. 1897).

In 1889, Murphy separated amicably from Dr. Lee and opened his own office. Although his practice was slow in getting started, from its beginning Murphy made sure it would have an academic flavor. He obtained an appointment as lecturer in surgery at Rush Medical College and he established an animal laboratory in a barn behind his house. As the volume of his surgery increased, he began lecturing whenever he operated, and soon visitors sought out his surgical theater. The keystones of his career were in place and in a remarkably short time (1892) he was made a professor of clinical surgery at the College of Physicians and Surgeons, which ultimately was to become the College of Medicine of the University of Illinois. Murphy was only thirty-five years of age.

Murphy was a controversial figure, to say the least. One can read damning criticism and flattering praise, but between these extremes one discerns a superb clinician, an engaging teacher, and a very skillful surgeon.

Franklin Martin found him "sensitive and reserved, admitting few to that inner man of quick human understanding, ready sympathy, worldly wisdom, keen humor, and boundless loyalty" (*SC* 591, p. 1000), while Sir W. Arbuthnott Lane remarked "there are few men who have ever attracted me as he did. He had a wonderful personality that made him the idol of American surgeons and endeared him to all" (*SC* 591, p. 998).

Murphy was also greatly admired by Paul Magnuson, who described him as "tall and straight behind his desk, the perfect picture of a doctor with his neatly parted gray beard, he looked out over the rims of polished half-moon glasses. You could be sure that life with John Benjamin Murphy would never be dull. His restless energy, flamboyant personality and superb technic, his daring trying the new and unorthodox, his personal feuds with half the other surgeons in town, combined to create an atmosphere of excitement" (3).

But not all of his biographers are so complimentary. One of Murphy's associates at Northwestern University, L. B. Arey, felt that "despite his greatness in many particulars, Dr. Murphy had a singular ability to arouse envy, distrust, and dislike. Even colleagues in the same hospital were not above spiteful whisperings. His scientific reports were alleged to suppress unfavorable cases. He was charged with being a social climber, a publicity seeker and a sensationalist. Certain it is that he had a talent for creating unfortunate publicity and headlines, and a positive genius for being misunderstood" (1). In contrast, Lord Moynihan claimed that "absolute truthfulness was the dominant expression of Murphy's personality . . . he never looked at truth askance or strangely" (5).

Moynihan also found him "an arresting personality. Even after the briefest intercourse with him there were only a few people who did not realize that he possessed a curious and subtle power of impressing a sense of his character upon them. His very handsome face, his tall, spare, almost gaunt figure, his high pitched and vibrant voice, his burning and quenchless enthusiasm for all of its manifold activities, his power of complete self-expression, all clamoured for notice, and caught and held the most eager attention" (5).

Deaver of Philadelphia agrees with Moynihan. "The influence of this towering personality was also felt in the broader fields of the medical world. He was a powerful, vigorous public speaker, full of enthusiasm and earnestness, which, coupled with a delightful personality and delightful humor, at once gained for him the attention of his hearers, young and old alike" (*SC* 591, p. 996).

Because of some of the negative reactions, Murphy had considerable trouble being elected to membership in the American Surgical

Association. Prewitt's comments before that group were considered by Ravitch (7) to be in reference to Murphy: "the self-laudatory egotist who seeks, after the manner of the charlatan, to impress upon an unenlightened and gullible public his superiority to all others, who covets the notoriety which the frequent appearance of his name in the public press may bring, must be persona non grata. . . ."

Murphy was often accused of self-promotion. His detractors objected especially to the considerable publicity that arose from his flamboyance in such episodes as the Haymarket Riot, the assassination attempt on Theodore Roosevelt, and the establishment of his new offices.

THE HAYMARKET RIOT

The Murphys had just returned from their honeymoon when the Haymarket Square Riot erupted. During a labor-related dispute, a bomb was thrown into a crowd of strikers and policemen in the square on the evening of May 4, 1886. Many of the bomb victims were taken to Cook County Hospital where they required operations. Murphy, then twenty-nine years old, was a staff surgeon at the hospital and operated on the injured all that night and into the next morning, outlasting other surgeons who succumbed to exhaustion.

A few months later, Murphy was asked to testify at the court trials of the alleged bomb throwers. The defense was trying to prove that the policemen, who had been arranged in two parallel lines, had shot each other with their revolvers. Murphy, to counter this argument, gave extensive descriptions of the nature of the injuries and of his operations in order to establish that the wounds resulted from bomb fragments rather than from pistol bullets (2).

The elements of this affair—an anarchist's bomb exploding at a labor union meeting, dead and dying policemen, and the young surgeon operating all night to save them—were all duly reported in the press, capturing the public's imagination. The graphic descriptions Murphy gave of his operations, while innocent on the surface, were resented by many of his surgical colleagues in Chicago, who saw them as no more than self-serving publicity.

He was accused of collusion in getting so many patients assigned to his service at Cook County Hospital, of collecting huge fees for his services, and of making derogatory remarks about his fellow surgeons when he was on the witness stand. There was never any evidence to support the more serious claims and Davis says, "from what we can

make out at this distance, Murphy's most dreadful sin was in drama-
tizing himself, in overplaying a scene." It was after this episode that
his practice gained considerably in volume.

THE ASSASSINATION ATTEMPT ON ROOSEVELT

Vice President Theodore Roosevelt became the twenty-sixth president
of the United Sates in 1901, following the assassination of William
McKinley. He served two terms and was succeeded by William
Howard Taft in 1909. In 1912, Roosevelt decided to try for yet another term and to challenge Taft for the nomination as the Republi-
can candidate for the coming election. The party became split between the two, and Roosevelt withdrew to establish a new
Progressive Party. When he declared that he felt as fit as a bull moose
the party acquired its nickname, the Bull Moose Party.

On October 14, 1912, Roosevelt arrived in Milwaukee to deliver a
campaign speech. As he waved from the car that was to take him to
the auditorium, he was struck in the right mid-chest by an assailant's
bullet. Not realizing that the candidate had been hit, the group started
to the auditorium. Then someone noticed a hole in Roosevelt's heavy
army overcoat. Roosevelt put his hand beneath his coat and found
blood on his shirt. It was later discovered that the bullet had penetrat-
ed not only the heavy coat but the thick folded notes for his speech
and a metal spectacle case before entering the flesh of his chest.

In spite of the bleeding, Roosevelt felt fine and insisted on going on
with the plans. He spoke for fifty minutes, letting his coat fall open to
reveal the blood on his shirt. After the speech, he was taken to the
emergency hospital where an roentgenogram revealed that the bullet
was lodged in the chest wall and that the lung was apparently unaf-
fected.

The first reaction was to send Roosevelt to Chicago, and various
people called four different Chicago surgeons: Arthur D. Bevan, L. L.
McArthur, Albert J. Ochsner, and John B. Murphy. Then the plan
was changed to bring the surgeons to Milwaukee instead of moving
the patient. The physicians were gathered at the railroad station for
the trip when yet another message came saying that the Bull Moose
would be brought to Chicago after all. The men agreed to reassemble
at the depot at 8:00 A.M.

It happened that Dr. Joseph Bloodgood from Johns Hopkins was
in Milwaukee and had insinuated himself into the proceedings. He
recommended to Roosevelt that only one surgeon be consulted and
that that surgeon should be Murphy (2). Roosevelt knew of Murphy's

fame and agreed. Accordingly, Bloodgood called the Murphy home and informed Mrs. Murphy of the decision and that the train would arrive about 5 A.M. When J. B. arrived at home from the depot, she gave him this information. At 5 A.M., Murphy was back at the train station with an ambulance and took the Bull Moose to Mercy Hospital.

Another version of the story has it that Murphy intercepted the train at a depot before the main station and spirited the patient away; yet another version claims that since Murphy was the surgeon for the railroad, he had the train diverted to the Navy Pier spur and he picked up the patient there (9).

The other surgeons assembled at the main station at 8:00 A.M., as had been agreed, before they discovered what had happened. Murphy did invite Bevan to consult but it seems he totally ignored McArthur and Ochsner.

At Mercy, another roentgenogram showed the bullet within the chest wall and the lung undamaged (fig. 1.1). Therefore, simple wound care was the only treatment and the bullet was never removed. The patient left the hospital on the eighth day.

During Roosevelt's hospital stay, Murphy released daily bulletins and also sent wires to the *New York Times*. In the bitter criticism that followed these incidents, Murphy was accused of stealing a patient and seeking publicity. Although formal complaints were registered with the American Medical Association, no decision was reached and no discipline was assessed.

MURPHY'S NEW OFFICES

By 1914, Murphy's practice was so large that anything that would improve efficiency was welcome. Obviously, the closer his office was to his hospital, the more convenient it would be. Immediately north of Mercy Hospital was a building called the Calumet Dispensary, which had been built in 1908 by Northwestern University as an outpatient teaching facility. Apparently the concept had not flourished so the building was sold for twenty thousand dollars to Murphy to be remodeled for his offices.

The architects did an excellent if somewhat lavish job, and there was great interest in the result on the part of physicians, as well as the public. Murphy was glad to oblige the press and the profession, and a great deal of publicity followed. (See figs. 1.2 through 1.6.) Even a volume of the *Surgical Clinics* contains an elaborate article on the new offices, including the floorplans and numerous photographs of the interior and of the physicians to whom Murphy rented space (*SC* 297). His ledgers list the names and the monthly payments of these renters. Sometime after Murphy's death this building reverted once again to an outpatient clinic called the Mercy Free Dispensary, which was used as a teaching facility by Mercy Hospital for Loyola University medical students until a new hospital opened in 1968.

The publicity surrounding the opening of Murphy's new offices elicited yet again a cry from Chicago physicians and surgeons that he was advertising unethically. Charges were brought to the American Medical Association, and at its meeting in San Francisco in July 1915 its Judicial Council reviewed the article and photographs. It found "the publication in question as being offensive and in bad taste, but because it was evident from the testimony that the publication complained of was not, in this instance, intended by the accused to be self-exploiting advertising, the Council accepted the defendant's explanation and apology" (8).

Davis (2) comments that

> the rest of the world might be fooled by John B. Murphy, but his enemies in Chicago thought they knew him for what he was: a sensationalist, an opportunist, a publicity seeker, and what newspapermen called "a trained seal"—a prominent person who is willing to be quoted on any subject at any time. They could concede that Murphy was something of a surgeon, indeed that he might have shown flashes of brilliance, but he was no conscientious healer, no mender of the maimed. He was interested purely and simply, they argued, in giving rein to his own ego—in doing the spectacular thing at a dramatic moment, in piling up a fortune, in climbing to the top in society, in publicizing himself to the housetops.

All this calumny occurred locally while Murphy was being acclaimed nationally and internationally, invited to speak at major meetings, made U.S. representative on important commissions, and honored in Europe. In hindsight, without any good evidence to support the accusations, it seems likely that much of this bitterness was instigated by envy of Murphy's obvious genius and by resentment of his arrogance.

On the basis of some of these claims, he was censured by the Chicago Medical Society and was refused membership for several years. Some of the censure reached the national scene and, as noted above, he had a great deal of difficulty getting elected to the American Surgical Association. His name was placed in nomination in 1895 but ta-

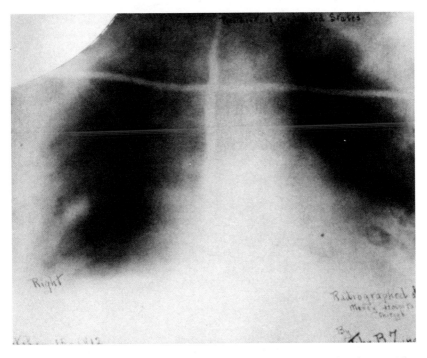

Fig. 1.1. A copy of the glass-plate X-ray of Theodore Roosevelt's thorax. The shadow of the bullet is barely visible in the lower left corner. The upper left corner of the plate has been broken off. The original plate hangs in Mercy Hospital, Chicago.

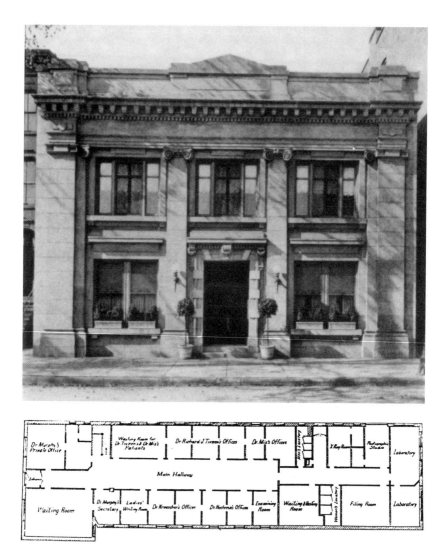

Fig. 1.2. Exterior and plan of Murphy's new offices next to Mercy Hospital.

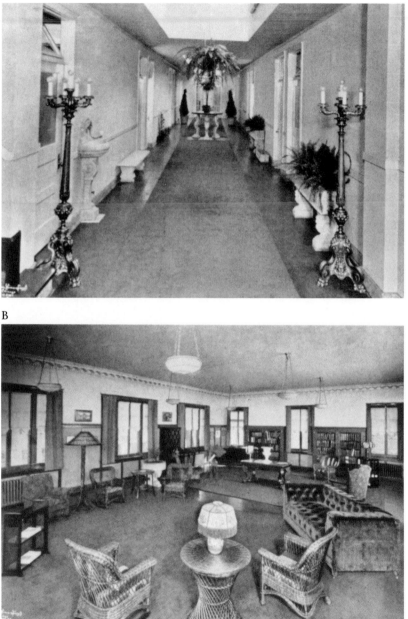

Fig. 1.3. Murphy's offices. (A) Main hallway on both sides of which the offices opened. (B) Library and lounge.

A

B

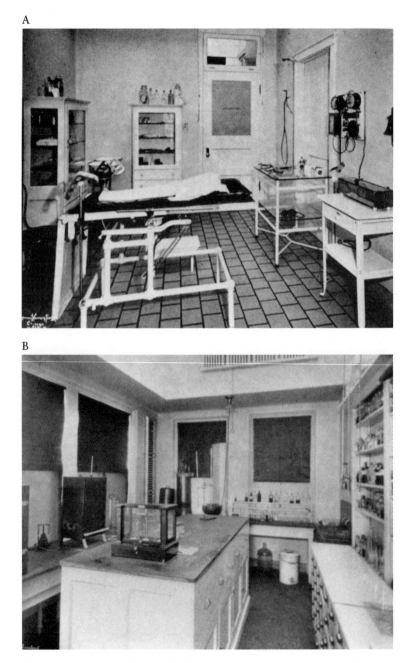

Fig. 1.4. Murphy's offices. (*A*) Examining and dressing room. (*B*) Laboratory, room no. 1.

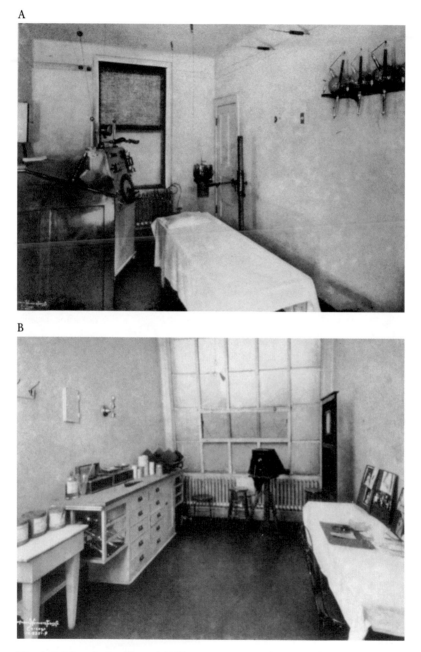

Fig. 1.5. Murphy's offices. (*A*) X-ray room. (*B*) Photographic studio where cases were photographed.

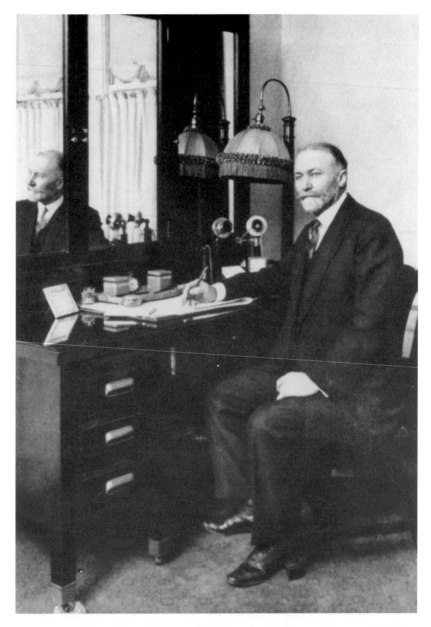

Fig. 1.6. Murphy in his office. Much of Murphy's office equipment, including the desk shown here, is on loan from the Sisters of Mercy to the Museum of Science and Industry in Chicago, which has a replica of his early office.

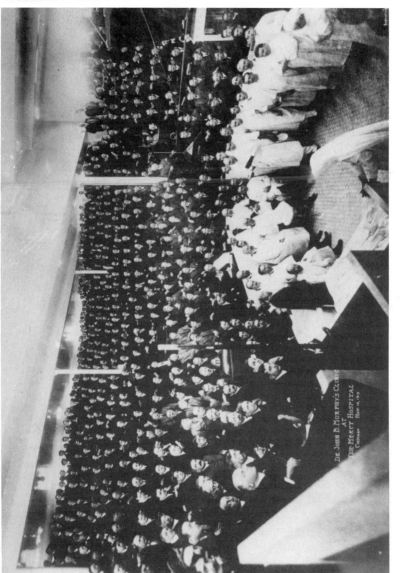

Fig. 1.7. The crowd in Murphy's Mercy Hospital amphitheater on November 12, 1913, during the Clinical Congress of Surgeons of North America.

bled. It was resubmitted in 1899 but voted down at the 1900 meeting. Finally, he was elected in 1902, but even then his early papers often went undiscussed.

In light of these difficulties and his being brought before the Judicial Council of the American Medical Association for similar complaints relating to his treatment of Theodore Roosevelt—for which no discipline was meted out—it is ironic that he later became president of the American Medical Association, the Chicago Medical Society, and the Chicago Surgical Society.

SCIENTIST, AUTHOR, TEACHER

Unique for his time, Murphy had his own animal laboratory. He recommended "for those of you who expect to follow surgery in practice let me outline a scheme of future study. First, plan to do regularly some experimental dog work, and do it with the same care that you would use on the human patient and with the same consideration for the feelings of the dog so far as pain is concerned; and after operation give the dog the same care as a patient. I have said of my dogs that they received as much nursing and attention as my patients" (*SC* 234, p. 410). He suggested starting with surgery on arteries and veins, since hemorrhage is so important to the surgeon, then on the lung and finally on the abdomen. Murphy almost always took a difficult problem to his laboratory before approaching it in the human patient.

In his first two homes the laboratory was in a barn behind the house, but in his third home it was a well-equipped, specially planned facility over the garage. This was a surprise gift from his wife, who also helped him there with animal care, anesthesia, and record keeping. His office records reveal that Mrs. Murphy transcribed many of his letters to patients and to referring doctors in her clear handwriting.

Murphy's writings are voluminous for the time (see Appendix A). If one counts the individual lectures in the *Surgical Clinics* in addition to the journal articles and book chapters, there are almost eight hundred separate items. In most pieces there are reviews of the literature, in-depth discussions of anatomy and physiology, citations of experimental work concerning the topic (including his own), and extensive presentation of clinical aspects and operative technics.

Many case reports are included in his writings, and the histories are given in great detail, especially in the *Surgical Clinics*. Off and on, the referring physicians are identified and those assisting at the operation are named. Occasionally some of the visitors in his operating room are mentioned—visitors such as William J. and Charles H. Mayo, George Crile, Nicholas Senn, Arthur Dean Bevan, Prince Albert of Monaco with his physician Louet, and other internationally prominent surgeons including Moynihan, Lane, Patterson, and Godlee.

He collected statistics worldwide, which he often referred to, especially in regard to the use of his anastomosis button and to the treatment of appendicitis. His files are replete with reprints, newspaper clippings (he subscribed to two clipping services), scribbled notes on the margins of programs from meetings he attended, and many drawings by medical artists that do not appear in any of his published articles. It may be that he was preparing a book on surgery at the time of his death.

Murphy was an outstanding teacher and his operative clinics were always well attended, commonly attracting one hundred to two hundred visitors. While he operated he lectured constantly in a high, strident voice. A secretary took down these remarks and eventually they were published in book form in *The Surgical Clinics of John B. Murphy at Mercy Hospital, Chicago*. His abilities in teaching led to numerous invitations from Chicago medical schools and hospitals and brought about several shifts in his institutional affiliations, as can be seen in his curriculum vitae.

Many famous visitors have described their reactions. Binnie recalls that

> as a clinical teacher Murphy had no peer. To watch the simple way in which he unraveled the history of a patient's ailments, eliminating the non-essentials, weighing the facts lest the apparently trivial should be really essential, and reducing the whole to an orderly story, was an intellectual treat. Then the systematic presentation of the results of his own examination of the patient, the comparison of these with the findings in other cases, a short discourse of the natural history of the disease in question and its proper treatment, were followed by a skillfully planned and executed operation, if such treatment was necessary. Large charts and lantern slide demonstrations were freely used to aid understanding. (*SC* 591, p. 992)

Moynihan agrees with Binnie, noting that "Murphy was beyond question the greatest clinical teacher of his day" (5), and George Crile says, "He taught the nurse, he taught the medical student, he taught the intern, he taught the young physician, he taught the veteran, he taught the laboratory worker, he taught the young surgeon, he taught the master surgeon, he taught the teachers of surgery. He taught the world" (*SC 591*, p. 993). And, finally, his admirer, Magnuson, comments that

> like all great teachers he had a magnificent streak of the theatrical in him. A noble figure in his long white gown, and with those penetrating eyes flashing over the rims of his gleaming half-moons, he made every movement a telling and dramatic one. The effect was heightened by his handsome regular features, his short cropped beard and mustache combed both ways from the middle, and above all the beautiful shape of his head, high and perfectly proportioned, its summit high-lighted by a gleaming bald spot across which he had his hair smoothly brushed from his right temple over towards the back of his left ear. (3)

THE AMERICAN COLLEGE OF SURGEONS

Milloy has recorded the details of Murphy's relationship to the American College of Surgeons (4). In 1904, a conversation between Murphy and Franklin H. Martin of Chicago resulted in the creation of a new surgical journal that was entitled *Surgery, Gynecology and Obstetrics,* which was to be directed more to the practical aspects of surgery rather than the theoretical. Murphy would become its editor in 1908.

Carrying the idea a step further, Martin decided to hold a "Clinical Congress of Surgeons of North America" in Chicago. At this congress visiting surgeons could observe operations at the various hospitals. Invitations were sent to all the subscribers of *SG&O* to attend the two-week meeting beginning November 7, 1910, and thirteen hundred accepted. There were subsequent annual meetings in Philadelphia and New York, and the popular success of these meetings led Martin to the concept of an American College of Surgeons to be modeled after the Royal College of Surgeons of England. What would have been the fourth meeting of the Clinical Congress, to be held in Chicago in November 1913, was scheduled to become the first meeting of the American College of Surgeons, with the initiation of nine hundred members. Because of the amalgamation of these two groups, the annual meetings subsequently became designated as gatherings of the Clinical Congress of the American College of Surgeons.

Earlier in 1913 Murphy, Harvey Cushing, Crile, and William Mayo had been made honorary members of the Royal College of Surgeons in London. At that time, they invited Sir Rickman Godlee, president of the Royal College, to give the inaugural address at the founding meeting of the American College of Surgeons. Godlee was described by Paget as the leading thoracic surgeon in Great Britain. While in Chicago for the opening ceremonies of the American College, he was the house guest of the Murphys. One wonders what discussions the two physicians might have had concerning the emerging field of thoracic surgery.

Murphy often invited visiting surgeons to speak or otherwise participate in his clinics. The week of November 10–15, 1913, during which many visitors were in Chicago for the inaugural meeting of the American College of Surgeons, is of particular interest. During that week he had as visiting speakers Dr. George Crile, founder of the Cleveland Clinic, and Dr. George Brewer from New York City, one of the twelve founders of the American College. Visitors from England, Mr. Patterson and Sir Rickman Godlee, also made remarks.

A volume of the *Surgical Clinics* (*SC 205*) lists the "Cases Operated on and Demonstrated by Dr. John B. Murphy at Mercy Hospital During the Week of the Clinical Congress of Surgeons of North America." This was the same week in which Murphy welcomed the distinguished speakers to his clinics. The article lists 149 patients; it is difficult to say how many were operated on for the visitors and how many were only demonstrated, but there were at least twenty operations including several arthroplasties, gallbladder operations, brain procedures, herniorrhaphies, and goiters. His operating amphitheater at Mercy Hospital was tightly filled on November 12 that week. There were some five hundred visitors in attendance (fig. 1.7).

After Murphy's death, many of his friends and family donated funds for the construction of the John B. Murphy Auditorium in Chicago, a magnificent structure that stands on the grounds of the American College of Surgeons at 55 East Erie Street. At the laying of the cornerstone of the auditorium on October 23, 1923, William J. Mayo said, "This is a fitting monument to the greatest surgeon of his day" (6).

CHRONOLOGY OF MURPHY'S LIFE

1857	Born in Appleton, Wisconsin, on December 21
1876	Graduated, Appleton High School
1879	Degree of Doctor of Medicine, Rush Medical College
1879–81	Intern, Cook County Hospital, Chicago
1881	Entered private practice

1882–84	Postgraduate studies, Vienna, Berlin, Heidelberg
1884	Back to private practice; appointed Lecturer in Surgery, Rush Medical College
1885	Married Jeanette C. Plamondon
1892	Professor of Clinical Surgery, College of Physicians and Surgeons (later the University of Illinois College of Medicine)
1892	Introduced the Murphy button for intestinal anastomosis
1895–1916	Chief of Surgery, Mercy Hospital, Chicago
1900–1916	President of Medical Staff, Mercy Hospital, Chicago
1901	Professor of Surgery, Northwestern University Medical School
1902	Awarded the Laetare Medal from the University of Notre Dame
1903	Vice-President, American Roentgen Ray Society
1905	Returned to Rush Medical College as Professor of Surgery
1905	President, Chicago Medical Society
1905	L.L.D., University of Illinois
1908	Returned to Northwestern as Professor of Surgery
1908	Master of Science, University of Sheffield, England
1910	President, Illinois State Medical Society
1911	President, American Medical Association
1913	President, Clinical Congress of Surgeons of North America, which that year established the American College of Surgeons
1913	Fellowship, Royal College of Surgeons of England
1915	L.L.D., Catholic University of America
1916	Died on 11 August at Mackinac Island, Michigan, while on vacation

REFERENCES

1. Arey, L. B., *Northwestern University Medical School 1859–1979* (Evanston: Northwestern University, 1979), 515.

2. Davis, L., *J. B. Murphy—Stormy Petrel of Surgery* (New York: Putnam, 1938).

3. Magnuson, P. B., *Ring the Night Bell* (Boston: Little, Brown, 1960), 72.

4. Milloy, F., "The contributions of John B. Murphy to thoracic surgery," *Surg. Gynecol. Obstet.* 171 (1990): 421–32.

5. Moynihan, B., "John B. Murphy—Surgeon," *Surg. Gynecol. Obstet.*

31 (1921): 549.

6. O'Regan, S. H., *Lord of the Knife* (Amherst, Wis.: Palmer, 1986), 14.

7. Ravitch, M. M., *A Century of Surgery* (Philadelphia: Lippincott, 1981), 209.

8. Rutkow, I. M., "A History of the Surgical Clinics of North America," *Surg. Clin. North Am.* 67 (1987): 1223.

9. Schmitz, R. L., "The Stormy Petrel and the Bull Moose," *Mercy Hospital Medical Center Journal* 4 (1987): 7.

2

MURPHY'S
PRACTICE IN GENERAL

*Robert L. Schmitz, Sr. Christeta Boring, and
Milorad M. Cupic*

In the latter half of the nineteenth century, when Murphy began his
career, American medical schools were in their infancy and the cur-
riculum consisted mainly of lectures. The two prominent schools in
Chicago were Rush Medical College and Chicago Medical College.
Physicians of note in the city included Christian Fenger, Edmund
Andrews, Nathan S. Davis, W. H. Byford, Ralph N. Isham, Nicholas
Senn, and Franklin H. Martin.

Medical science was still quite primitive. Patent medicines were ev-
erywhere. The armamentarium consisted largely of bloodletting, plas-
ters, emetics, and purging. Epidemics were common and the plagues
of malaria, cholera, and smallpox were being overtaken by those of
typhoid fever, tuberculosis, and syphilis. The germ theory of disease
was not widely accepted, although better sanitary conditions were
being recognized as important in controlling disease.

In spite of the new knowledge of anesthesia, surgery had remained
limited largely to amputations for trauma and cutting for bladder
stones. However, with the increasing acceptance of Lister's work and
by applying antiseptic precautions, surgeons found that it was becoming feasible to enter the abdomen without a prohibitive risk to the
patient, and the first nephrectomies, gastrectomies, and esophagec-
tomies were being done. The time was ripe for "The Century of the
Surgeon," as Thorwald (2) has named it, and for Murphy to come on
the scene.

Murphy's accomplishments can be better appreciated when they
are seen in the context of some of the important medical events that
occurred just before and during his life:

1842–46	Use of ether anesthesia by Long and Morton
1847	Use of chloroform by Simpson
1860	Lister's carbolic acid spray
1861	First nephrectomy by Wolcott
1879–81	Pean, Rydygier, and Billroth: first gastrectomies
1872	First esophagectomy by Billroth
1876	First Porro cesarian section
1878	Iodoform first used as an antiseptic
1886	Reginald Fitz described and named appendicitis
1887–88	Morton did the first two planned appendectomies
1890	Rubber gloves introduced by Halsted
1891	Halsted described his radical mastectomy
1895	Roentgen discovered the X-ray
1898	The Curies discovered radium

The primitive state of the art makes Murphy's contributions all the more noteworthy.

Early in his career, influenced by Moses Gunn and Christian Fenger, Murphy decided to specialize in surgery, and as soon as he could, he started animal operations and cadaver dissection. He already had qualms about the occasional operator or family doctor doing surgery, calling such physicians pseudo-surgeons. He wrote:

> I wish to emphasize the importance of technical training in operative work if you intend to practice surgery. The tinsmith, the shoemaker, the carpenter, have to devote many months and years of their time to the mechanical part of their art to train their hands to execute rapidly, systematically and concisely the various parts of their trade, while the pseudo-surgeon is so adept, so nimble-fingered, so superior that he can undertake the most complicated operation not only without having performed it on the cadaver or the lower animal, but without having seen or carefully read a description of the operation. (JBM 46, p. 202)

Soon after Murphy began his practice in 1884 it acquired a rapid tempo that only accelerated as time went on. By 1889 he had done his first appendectomy and was preaching that early operation was the solution to the high mortality rate from appendicitis. By 1892 he had switched from Rush to the College of Physicians and Surgeons, had advanced to the rank of professor of clinical surgery, and had introduced his anastomotic button.

This was the state of his practice and his career when he was invited to Mercy Hospital by Sister Raphael McGill in 1895 to consider a position as chief of surgery. At the time, Mercy was affiliated with Northwestern University and only its faculty members could operate at the hospital. Murphy accepted the appointment and therefore had to shift his school connection yet again. It proved a good move since by 1901 he had risen to the rank of professor of surgery at Northwestern. From 1895 until his death in 1916, he dominated Mercy Hospital's surgical service. On any given operating day, there were one hundred to two hundred visitors in his amphitheater, and by 1901 the hospital had to enlarge the amphitheater to accommodate the overflow crowds.

Among Murphy's papers are logs of operations done at Mercy Hospital from 1904 through 1908. A sampling of three hundred consecutive operations gives the following proportions of types of procedures that were done:

General Surgery	55%
Gynecology	10%
Neurosurgery	5%
Orthopedics	22%
Urology	7%
Others	1%

THE PATIENT

Murphy always stressed the details of the medical anamnesis and often pointed out that the diagnosis could be predicted from a careful interrogation. "Listen, listen to the patient's story! He is telling you the diagnosis," he said. Time and again in the *Surgical Clinics* write-ups there are notes of his cross-examination of the student or the intern over the details of the history; he continued to question until he got the data he wanted. On the basis of these he would predict what the findings would be at the operation.

Particular emphasis was given to several features of the history: 1) the menses, their timing and character; 2) any trauma, since he thought it was a factor in breast and bone cancer, as well as being of obvious significance in general; and 3) the order in which pain, nausea, and vomiting occurred in abdominal ailments.

One day Murphy said to his audience, "The most valuable portion of my medical experience has been derived, I believe, from the fact that during all these years of my practice, and in spite of the not inconsiderable labor which it involves, I have not only seen, but also examined carefully, practically every patient on whom I have expected to operate. That is my system" (*SC* 282, p. 932).

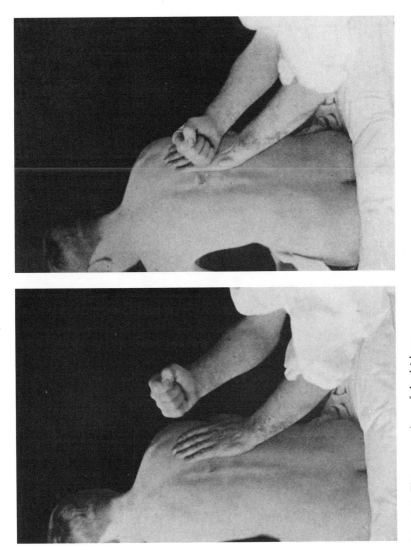

Fig. 2.1. Fist percussion of the kidney.

A

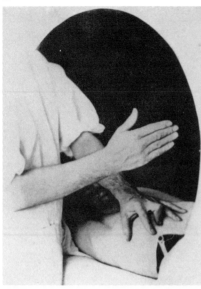

B

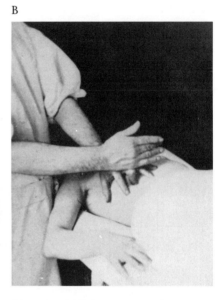

C

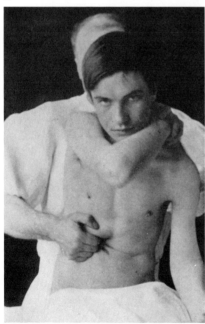

Fig. 2.2. (*A, B*) Hammer-stroke percussion of the gallbladder. (*C*) Deep-grip palpation of the gallbladder.

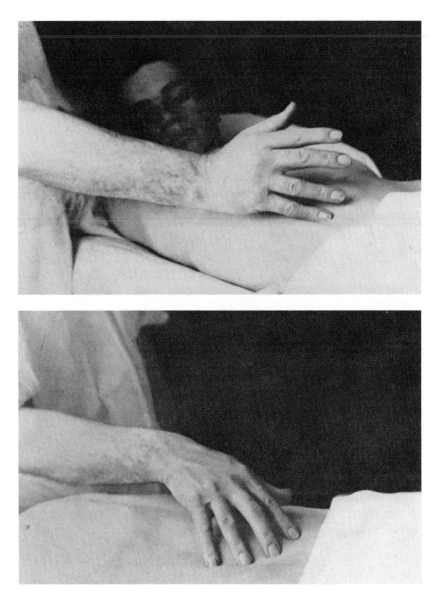

Fig. 2.3. Piano percussion.

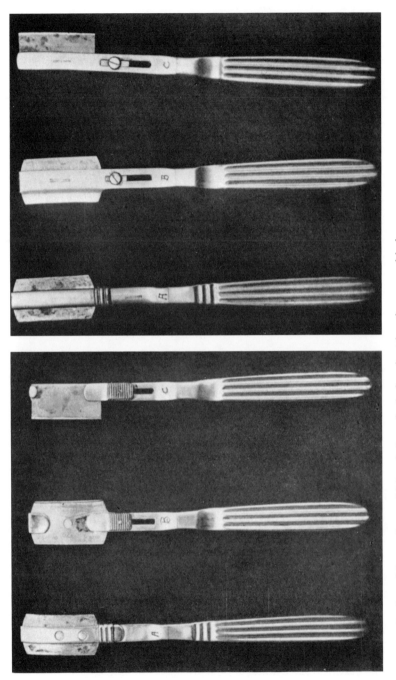

Fig. 2.4. Back and front views of Murphy's scalpels fitted with safety razor blades.

There are five maneuvers commonly used in the physical examination that bear Murphy's eponym; they are well illustrated with photographs in *Surgical Clinics* 52.

Murphy described fist percussion of the kidney (fig. 2.1):

> When the patient is suffering from an acute obstruction from any cause to the outlet of the ureter, or when the patient is suffering from an infarct in the kidney which increases the tension in its capsule, we can demonstrate that the lesion is in the kidney and not in the appendix, and not in the gallbladder, by fist percussion over the spine. Have the patient sit on the side of the bed, or on a chair, and stoop slightly or lean over forward. Place the left hand first over the supposedly normal kidney, and bring the fist down on it, striking a strong blow. There is no response; no manifestation of pain. Change the hand to the diseased side, press firmly against the site of the kidney, and make the fist percussion, and the patient springs up suddenly and sometimes cries out. It is one of the most pronounced responses that I know of to physical tests of diseases inside the wall of the abdomen. (SC 69, pp. 630–33)

In the second maneuver, hammer-stroke percussion of the gallbladder (fig. 2.2), the middle finger of the examiner's left hand is bent at a right angle and placed just below the mid-right costal arch of the patient; the patient is instructed to take a deep breath and as he does the examiner's right hand is used to deliver hammerlike blows to the dorsum of his left hand. If the gallbladder is tender, the patient reports acute pain in the abdomen.

The third maneuver, deep-grip palpation of the gallbladder (fig. 2.2), requires the examiner to stand at the patient's right and curl the fingers of his right hand upward behind the right costal margin; the patient is instructed to take a deep breath. If the gallbladder is tender, he will be unable to do so.

Piano percussion of the abdomen for fluid (fig. 2.3) is the fourth maneuver. The fingers are gently rippled in sequence on the abdominal wall; when fluid is present, even in small amounts, the usual tympanitis is replaced with a flat note.

The fifth maneuver is simultaneous palpation of the iliac fossae: The technique is used to pick up the difference in resistance between the two sides when inflammation of the appendix is present.

Included in Murphy's lectures to students are some he called "Murphy's Clinical Talks on Surgical and General Diagnosis." They are scattered through volumes 3 and 4 of the *Surgical Clinics*. Some of the subjects covered were empyema, tubal pregnancy, breast tumors, gastric and duodenal ulcers, carcinoma of the stomach, appendicitis, cholecystitis, ascending urinary infection, ileus, fibroids, renal and ureteral stone, hematuria, intrathoracic sarcoma, meningitis, perinephritic abscess, fracture dislocation of the spine, and Hodgkin's disease.

Murphy's aim was always to establish the diagnosis as accurately as possible, and he often went through an elaborate differential in front of his audience of students or visiting doctors before making his choice.

CANCER

Murphy treated a good many patients with cancer. He accepted the belief current at the time that it was caused by an infectious agent, perhaps a parasite, and/or trauma. As far as he was concerned the trauma need not be severe and a single episode, not sufficient to produce a laceration or fracture, could cause cancer in bone, breast, or testes. The disease began in an organ and spread to lymph "glands" by regional lymphatic routes and to the lungs, liver, and bone via the bloodstream. He considered all cancers to be equally virulent and any differences in clinical behavior he attributed to the host's resistance to the disease. Therefore, he doubted that early diagnosis would improve survival.

He felt that cancer was more frequent in the neck of organs, e.g., cervix, pylorus, urinary bladder, and gallbladder, because of the richer lymphatic supply at those points.

Murphy used frozen section diagnosis while operating but advised "never give a pathologist a report of what you think a tumor is. Get his weight of evidence as he interprets what he sees; then you add his findings and your clinical experience together and arrive at a diagnosis" (SC 24, p. 190).

Several times he mentioned "aneurysmal sarcomas" in the thymus, the bone, and the spinal canal, which bled profusely if manipulated. He advised against any attempt to remove them. A micrograph illustration (SC 168, p. 693) suggests these tumors were angiosarcomas.

He noted, "Remember, cancer in thin people metastasizes slower and grows slower both in the original primary location and in the metastases than it does in fat people." It is the thin patient that "gives the larger percentage of cures" (SC 204, p. 1082).

Within a year of Roentgen's report of his discovery of the X-ray, Murphy tried X-ray therapy. "Being interested, in common with other physicians and surgeons, in everything that promised to aid in the relief of suffering humanity, I, on June 8, 1896, referred to Dr. H. P. Pratt, who was then experimenting therapeutically with the X-rays, a case of lupus, suggesting that he experiment with this form of tuberculosis rather than the pulmonary form. The case was cured. This was I believe, the first case of lupus to be cured by X-rays" (JBM 64).

Various advanced cancers were also referred by him for radiation therapy and in one of them he recovered the breast after it had been irradiated. He says that

> it was very instructive. First, because of the fact that the ray reduced the size of this large mass (the size of an ink-well) to one two-and-a-half centimeters wide and four centimeters long. Second, because of the changes in the tumor itself. We sectioned it and when we came to examine the microscopic specimen we found that the changes were of two kinds: first, an increase in the connective tissue; second, a decrease in the cellular elements of the carcinoma. . . . The cells showed vacuolization, but the nucleus did not seem to be changed at all. . . . Another interesting feature was the fact that the glands (lymph nodes) had not changed the least. (JBM 64)

In discussing a report by P. S. O'Donnell, he claims another first. He referred to him a pregnant woman with an unusual physical finding. "I conceived the idea of having a skiagram made, and sent the patient at once to Dr. O'Donnell. This is the first time the idea of making a skiagram of the fetus in utero had been suggested to him" (JBM 119).

The glimmerings of modern chemotherapy may be seen in Murphy's use of arsenicals in advanced malignancies, e.g., bone (*SC* 550; 593, p. 1037) and ovary (*SC* 78, p. 711; 252, p. 609).

MURPHY'S OPERATING THEATER

Murphy was an early advocate of Listerian antisepsis and fought for it vigorously in Chicago and in Mercy Hospital. He felt that the nuns who worked in the operating rooms should wear white rather than the customary black, and he worked with Sister Raphael, the hospital administrator, to get the necessary permission from the Vatican.

Each evening before an operating day, Murphy held a planning session with Sister Victorine or Sister Ludwina, his scrub nurses. Together they discussed the order of the operations, any special instruments needed, and any special precautions to be observed.

On one occasion he turned to his assistant and asked, "Where has this patient been marked? We do not want to take out the wrong side, an accident which is very frequent. Remember, the wrong eye has been taken out, the wrong leg has been amputated, the wrong Gasserian ganglion has been removed, and the wrong side has been operated on for hernia because of a lack of system in marking. If you have a system, that is what counts and saves trouble" (*SC* 74, p. 686).

Murphy's abdominal-wound closure was always the same: "The peritoneum is closed with a continuous catgut suture, everting the edges, making an ectropion, so that there will be no raw surface in the peritoneal cavity. That will prevent the formation of adhesions. Next we insert figure-of-8 stitches of silkworm-gut, completely obliterating all dead spaces. The skin-edges are approximated with horsehair, making a continuous suture. The wound is then dusted with a bismuth subiodid, a desiccating powder, not an antiseptic, and sealed with a collodion gauze dressing" (*SC* 72, p. 671). (The senior editor of this book had exactly this closure after an appendectomy at Mercy Hospital, Chicago, in 1929 by one of Murphy's pupils, Edward Kelly. He also remembers well the "piano percussion" of the abdomen during the preoperative evaluation by an internist, Robert Berghoff.)

There was a sponge count after each case and the hospital record included a reference to its correctness:

> Let the record show that Sister Ludwina reports the sponges counted and correct; that on the first count one sponge was missing, but that it was found rolled up in another sponge. Let the record further show that the operator made a careful inspection of the field to determine that no sponges or instruments were left.
>
> We have lost only one sponge since we started to keep a systematic count of them, and that one was never accounted for. We do know that it was not left in the patient. We lost one other sponge in an operation on the bladder. We reopened the bladder at once and demonstrated that it was not there. Then we found it later in the hallway just outside the amphitheater. It must have stuck to someone's shoe and thus was carried out (*SC* 285).

The events of each operation were dictated to a secretary present in the operating room, often prefaced with the phrase "Let the record show." The record included the history, what was done at the operation, and many side remarks referring to the literature and to cases of a similar nature that he had previously encountered.

Murphy experimented with a gutta-percha solution to coat the hands as a substitute for rubber gloves, which he felt impeded his touch (JBM 80); he said in a second report (JBM 83) that he was using it exclusively, but there was no further mention of it and he seems to have given it up.

Since scalpels were often dull, he modified regular scalpel handles so that single- or double-edged razor blades could be attached. He related, "I have used these for some time in all my work and have found them very serviceable and satisfactory" (JBM 121; SC 85) (see fig. 2.4). Whether or not he continued to use them throughout his career is not clear. He devised or modified numerous other instruments for his own preferences in various operations. (These are mentioned in the appropriate chapters of this book.)

In contrast to the highly technological delivery of anesthesia today, materials available in the early 1900s were relatively crude. Murphy had a choice of ether, chloroform, or nitrous oxide used in combination with ether and/or oxygen. The administration was usually by the "open system" using a wire-framed, gauze-covered (Esmarch) mask; however, in an operation for carcinoma of the lip, he mentioned using a nasal tube to deliver ether vapor (SC 64, p. 575), and he did "believe that hernias in the aged should be operated with a local anesthetic" (SC 67, p. 627). He noted, too, "In all laparotomy, goiter, and brain cases oxygen should be given during the general anesthetic" (SC 67, p. 628).

Murphy used ether almost exclusively because he considered it much safer than chloroform, in spite of ether's inflammability. In discussing anesthesia with his audience, he recounted:

This recalls the unpleasant experience I had with chloroform, where I kept up artificial respiration for three hours and fifteen minutes. I went over to let water flow on my hands, turned around, and saw a change in the patient's face. In thirty seconds she was apparently dead. Her heart had stopped beating, her respiration had stopped, and she was for all intents and purposes dead. We started artificial respiration, then we resorted to dilatation of the rectum. When the rectum ceased to respond to rhythmic dilatation for six or eight minutes, her respiratory center being out of commission, we went to the upper sphincter of the sigmoid, put our thumbs away up, and ten times in a minute we would dilate to see if she would make an effort at inspiration. The heart kept on doing its work, the pallor diminished, but the minute we stopped dilating respiration ceased. We changed to the vagina, dilated that ten times in a minute, and we kept that up until she finally started in voluntary respiration.

Her pulse was 200 the next day, but with care and watching closely she got well. (*SC* 67, p. 626)

His anesthetic services were supplied by a nursing nun, Sister Ethelreda, "a mistress of her art" who he said delivered fifteen thousand to sixteen thousand anesthesias over a thirteen-year period without an anesthetic death (*SC* 67). Sister Christeta Boring at Mercy Hospital says that it is quite possible that Sister Ethelreda, who worked in surgery every day, could have given twenty-five to thirty anesthetics a week, which would support Murphy's statement quoted above.

It was Murphy's requirement that the patient be seen by the anesthetist the evening before surgery to check on the clinical status and the laboratory reports in the chart and that these be discussed with the surgeon in advance of the operation. The patient was to be carefully prepared for the induction, monitored throughout the operation, and then "assisted in coming out of the anesthetic." Premedication consisted of morphine and atropine. "We are firm believers in the advantages of atropin. . . . it very materially lessens secretion" (*SC* 67).

Murphy described the process of induction: "The anesthetic is begun with gas (nitrous oxide). When the patient begins to lose consciousness, the change is made from gas to ether, which is given with an Esmarch mask by the drop method. When anesthesia is complete, just sufficient ether is given to maintain sleep" (*SC* 67, p. 628). Even without the multiple drugs and the numerous machines available to administer anesthesia today, Murphy was cognizant of the importance of anesthesia to the outcome of surgical procedures and saw that it was attended to properly.

Murphy liked to teach at the operating table and in the amphitheater, and some of his visitors have left us their impressions. Sir Rickman Godlee found:

The morning clinics at the hospital were times never to be forgotten. The theater was crowded from floor to ceiling with an enthusiastic audience. . . . The rush to obtain the coveted places showed how his professional brethren appreciated his method of instruction. . . . It was evident that he was putting his whole soul into his teaching. He made the most simple subjects exciting, and the most abstruse subjects clear. The didactic style, the word-play with the unfortunate intern, the copious diagrams, and the display of skiagrams kept all his hearers on the alert, and the speed and direction of his operations and the demonstration of successful results were a source of admiration and envy. (*SC* 591, p. 996)

In a similar vein Lord Moynihan wrote:

There he stood in the middle of the circle, in the theater, with his assistants and friends in the first row, and the other benches packed to the roof with eager students, or with medical men, who came again and again to learn from him afresh. As he began to speak one felt a strange sense of disappointment, and even dismay. For while the handsome face and upright figure were things of real beauty, the voice in which he began to speak was quite unpleasant. It was harsh, even raucous, high pitched, shrill, apt to wander into other keys. . . . But as he continued to speak the voice gradually ceased to distract, it became smoother, quieter, and more evenly pitched, and all thought of it was now lost in the rapt attention to the matter. . . . And then Murphy would operate. . . . Every step in every operation which I ever saw him do was completed deliberately, accurately, once for all. It led inevitably to the next step, without pause, without haste; that step completed, another followed. And so when the end came, a review of the operation showed no false move, nor part left incomplete, no chance of disaster; all was honest, sage and simple; it was modest rather than brilliant. (1)

A picture that several authors have painted is described by an unidentified editor of the *Surgical Clinics of North America:*

No one who has been present will ever forget the manner in which, at the conclusion of an operation, and while the patient was being rolled out and the next patient prepared and brought in, Dr. Murphy was wont to seat himself upon a stool in the center of the arena, and, surrounded by the big family of visiting physicians and surgeons from the far corners of the earth, discourse to them at great length upon the salient features of the operation just finished, correlating similar cases from his vast personal experience. He sat leaning forward cross-legged on the stool, and with elbow on knee, in full operating regalia, earnest, decisive, and incisive, talking in a clear and forceful manner, with a well-modulated though high-pitched voice, and keeping his big family-circle spellbound by his eloquent word-pictures. (Editor's note, *SC* 591, p. 986)

After this general overview, we are ready to examine specific details of Murphy's surgical practice. The following chapters will discuss his approaches to general surgery, gynecology, neurosurgery, orthopedics, thoracic surgery, urology, vascular surgery, and infectious diseases.

REFERENCES

1. Moynihan, B., "John B. Murphy—Surgeon," *Surg. Gynecol. Obstet.* 31 (1920): 549.

2. Thorwald, J., *The Century of the Surgeon* (New York: Pantheon, 1957).

3

GENERAL SURGERY

*William A. Tito, William H. Blair, and
Alejandra Perez-Tamayo*

In the early 1900s patients often presented late in the course of disease. Without the availability of aggressive resuscitative technics, expeditious diagnostic tests, perioperative antibiotics, blood transfusions, and refined anesthetic practices, mortalities were frequent.

APPENDICITIS

In 1886, a hallmark paper presented by Reginald H. Fitz (Boston) clearly described the pathology of appendicular inflammation and its sequelae (5). He recommended removal of the inflamed appendix and pointed out that frequent abscesses in the right iliac fossa were not due to typhlitis, perityphlitis, paratyphlitis, or epityphlitis, but to perforation of the appendix. Fitz coined the term appendicitis to describe this condition.

In the following year (1887) Thomas Morton—son of William Morton, who discovered ether anesthesia—performed the first successful removal of an appendix (12). He had a great deal of motivation in his act since he had lost a brother and a son to appendicitis that had been treated conservatively. He performed the operation on a twenty-six-year-old male who had a long history of attacks. At surgery Morton observed that the appendix had already perforated. The patient survived.

On March 2, 1889, J. B. Murphy intentionally operated "early" on a patient with appendicitis with the aim of excising the organ before rupture had occurred; he opened a new epoch in surgery. K. A. Meyer of Chicago and W. W. Musgrove of Canada (13) claimed that this was the first time that an appendectomy was deliberately planned prior to rupture of the organ. Harold Ellis, however, claims that Robert Lawson Tait in 1880 "was the first to diagnose and successfully remove an acutely inflamed appendix" (4).

Herrick (7) remembered transferring this "first" patient to Murphy's ward at Cook County Hospital and said it was case #2 in Murphy's paper in the *JAMA* (JBM 19). In that same paper was recorded the drainage of a perityphlitic abscess by Murphy in November 1885, a year before Fitz's epic paper. The importance of these events cannot be overemphasized. The surgery of appendicitis was now on a new footing. Attack prior to rupture would prevent the complications that resulted in the usual disastrous mortality rate of the disease.

Following this beginning, Murphy campaigned for early operation for appendicitis, a stance contrary to the prevailing view that this disease should only be treated by medical means. Murphy stated that "removal of the appendix at the first signs of inflammation was the way to a permanent cure" (JBM 23).

Said Murphy:

> The mention of "expectant treatment" for appendicitis is like the waving of the banderillo's red scarf at el toro. I can't keep quiet. I am still hunting for a term which expresses my opinion of the method. I find the English vocabulary too limited, however, to suit my desires. A Latin medicus might have called it the expectans mortem treatment. To name it the manana method is not malapropos, but it is too mild. To describe it as dolce far niente is expressive, but this soft Italian phrase is impossible when I am showing all my teeth in a Rooseveltian glare. If I had Roosevelt's genius for phraseology I might find the needed term, but as yet it eludes me. (*SC* 313, p. 5).

At that time the usual late surgical approach in the treatment of appendicitis produced about the same mortality as medical treatment, approximately 30 percent. The mortality with perforation and diffuse peritonitis was over 85 percent. By 1895 Murphy had reported on 207 patients on whom he had electively operated with an overall mortality of 10 percent (JBM 13; 16; 19; 23; 26; 35). By 1904 he had performed 2,000 appendectomies with less than a 2 percent mortality (JBM 77). The battle for early operation was being won.

The argument over which treatment was correct raged for many years. Murphy was the leader of the early operation concept, which eventually prevailed, but many others contributed to his success story. Of particular importance were Charles McBurney, the Mayo brothers, and A. J. Ochsner. Ochsner was particularly important since he resolved the best method of treating post-ruptured appendices, that is, starvation, hot stupes, and elevation of the upper torso (Fowler Position) with elective removal of the appendix at a later date.

Murphy's technique for appendectomy should be recounted:

> I want to show you how to cover the mesentery. . . . I will pass my needle through one layer on the right, then on through the layer on the left, and then come back and make an overstitch. The overstitch first ligates the vessels, then comes through and approximates that peritoneum from both sides. Now I have a continuous circle of peritoneum for primary adhesions. We have from the beginning considered the opening made by amputating the appendix the same as a bullet wound of the intestine, and we close it with exactly the same precautions.
>
> We are back to the starting-point of that stitch. It is not pulled taut. . . . We now put in the puckering-string suture in the base of the caput coli, the appendix stump being in the center of the loop of the suture.
>
> You will have noticed how I pushed the infective contents of the appendix upwards with the hemostat. I milked it up, and then ligated the appendix in the line where I crushed it with the hemostat. I want to keep the forceps on the appendix until we make a smear and culture of its contents, and also from its wall. Then I amputated it and touched the stump with 95 per cent phenol. I do not neutralize it, because I am going to turn it in, and it will take care of itself. The next step is to pull taut the purse-string suture and invert the appendix. . . . Now we have closed the intestine. (*SC* 106, p. 113)

CALCULOUS GALLBLADDER DISEASE

In Murphy's time, autopsy findings suggested that 10 percent of adults had gallstones, and that approximately 10 percent of these had symptoms attributable to stones. Thus the prevalence of symptomatic cholelithiasis was 1 percent of the general population. Antisepsis was in its infancy and no practical antibiotics were available for patients with cholecystitis. Operations of the day included cholecystoenterostomy, cholecystostomy, cholecystectomy, and cholecystendysis. Such procedures carried significant morbidity and high mortality rates. Even more morbidity was incurred if the common duct needed incision.

Murphy wrote:

> You will find in reviewing results of operations that mortality is greatest in the operation of cholecystenterostomy, in one sitting, by means of suture, in which thirty-five percent of the cases terminated fatally. The operation showing the next greatest fatality is cholecystendysis, with a mortality of twenty-three percent. Next high in the scale of mortality is cholecystostomy, in one sitting, the operation which is most prevalent and performed more frequently than any other, and almost as frequently as all the others combined; its mortality is nineteen percent. (JBM 18)

Murphy drew from the experience of Courvoisier that cholecystitis evolved with colic and suppurative changes. He advocated a physical examination that elicited parietal irritation (Murphy's sign). Because most symptomatic patients treated medically would deteriorate, since there were no antibiotics, Murphy championed early operation. In 1882, Carl Langenbuch had introduced cholecystectomy, but mortality rates ran high unless there were few adhesions and the anatomy was favorable for the surgeon. Therefore, without antibiotics and blood transfusions for support, the usual operation was a quick bypass procedure. Indeed, if the choledochus was obstructed, such bypasses facilitated more favorable outcomes.

Murphy said, "I am very much in favor of cholecystectomy where it is practicable, but the number of cases in which it is feasible is very limited, even much more than those for cholecystenterostomy. Where the gallbladder is sufficiently long and the adhesions are limited, we can do the operation of cholecystectomy very well, but this operation is contraindicated when the adhesions are extensive, as it is when there has been recent jaundice. When there is occlusion of the common duct you do not benefit your patient by this operation" (JBM 25).

Because of such reasoning Murphy preferred cholecystenterostomy in most of his gallbladder operations and it was this preference that led to the development of his anastomotic button.

When the gallbladder was too inflamed even for bypass, Murphy would do only a cholecystostomy and remove what stones were accessible. In one such patient, before removing the drain permanently, he inserted a cystoscope through the drain site into the gallbladder and removed a residual stone with a hook passed through the cystoscope (SC 48).

THE MURPHY BUTTON

The difficulties inherent in anastomosis within the digestive tract plagued surgeons for centuries. Attempts to solve this problem followed two tracks: the development of suture technics and the invention of mechanical devices.

There were two major stumbling blocks in the path of the development of suture methods to join the bowel: it was believed that reaction to the suture material might obliterate the lumen and that the way to approximate the cut edges was to join the mucous layer of the one side to the serous layer of the other.

The first real progress in suture anastomosis was the demonstration by Joubert and Lembert that good bowel union will follow if the serous surfaces are approximated. Eventually it was established that two things had to be done: 1) serosa had to be apposed to serosa to produce a seal against intestinal leakage; 2) the suture "bites" had to traverse the sero-muscular layer in order to hold the union. But until these principles were learned, anastomosis of bowel by suture technic was hazardous.

In 1826, at the time Joubert and Lembert were working with sutures, Denens developed a technic of intestinal anastomosis utilizing hollowed silver tubes. He forced a hollowed tube into each cut end of the bowel so that the edges were inverted and joined the bowel together by adding a third tube into the previously inserted tubes. Sutures were placed into the bowel over the tubes. With this device he achieved cut end inversion with serosa-to-serosa contact and mechanical approximation. Unfortunately, the pressure from the metal tubes caused tissue necrosis and perforation.

In 1887 Nicholas Senn, a Chicago surgeon, developed an anastomosis technic utilizing hollow bone plates to join the bowel together. The bone plates were placed into the bowel lumen and then stitched together. But they, too, led to perforation and obstruction.

Since all approaches to date had a high failure rate, the time was ripe for a better solution to the problem. As Murphy was wont to do, he took the enigma to his laboratory and experimented on canines. He established to his satisfaction that two serosal surfaces brought together will unite by adhering and that living tissue compressed between two surfaces will slough away, leaving a scar that is not likely to contract.

From this work he developed his button. This device consisted of two metal circular rings, one with a male tube protruding through the ring and the other with a female receptor. The buttons (rings) were placed in the lumen of the divided bowel ends to be joined and held by a purse-string suture. The purse string inverted the cut edges and placed the serosa outwardly. After the suture placement, the rings were attached by pushing the threaded male tube into the female tube, which had a spring catch to hold the two parts. The device was self-retaining and offered an adequate lumen until it sloughed and passed out with defecation (figs. 3.1 and 3.2).

Murphy's first use of the button experimentally was to join the gallbladder directly to the upper part of the small intestine to relieve biliary obstruction. The first animal surgery was done in early June 1892, and in December of that year Murphy reported in the *Medical Record* (JBM 15) on the results of his animal experiments. He emphasized several features of button approximation: 1) the button retained its position approximation; 2) ideal apposition of the surfaces was achieved; 3) there were no sutures at the anastomosis site; 4) upon healing, a linear scar was produced with minimal constricture; and 5) the extreme simplicity of the technic and speed of placement reduced operative morbidity. By this time, he had used the button successfully in many types of procedures including end-to-end and side-to-side intestinal anastomosis and gastroenterostomy. Invariably the buttons passed by the eighteenth day postoperatively.

Six months after the first animal experiments, the button was used in a human patient. Over time, Murphy fashioned 334 biliary bypasses using the button with minimal operating time and an operative mortality reduced by a factor of ten. The development of complications such as mechanical bowel obstruction predicted by Nicholas Senn never materialized. While some patients remained symptomatic from chronic cholecystitis, none suppurated from unabated obstruction. Murphy's solution was replaced only after significant advances could be made in anesthesia, perioperative resuscitation, and improved suture technique.

It was claimed that Murphy could implant the button for cholecystoenterostomy in eleven to eighteen minutes. When cholecystostomy seemed a safer operation, Murphy used the button to connect the gallbladder directly to the abdominal wall; if the gallbladder would not reach, he put an extension tube on the button (figs. 3.3 and 3.4).

Before the introduction of the Murphy button there were only eleven cases on record in which attempts were made to join the gallbladder to the intestines for relief of biliary obstruction. At the same time only forty-seven operations to remove the gallbladder had been successful; it was a very hazardous undertaking.

In April 1893, Dr. Charles Mayo visited Murphy's clinic and for the first time saw an operation performed with the button. Later that month Dr. William Mayo successfully placed a Murphy button between the gallbladder and duodenum of a seventy-one-year-old male with biliary obstruction and jaundice (2). Following that, the use of the button was commonplace at the Mayo Clinic until 1935 when suture methods superseded it.

Prior to the use of the button, successful anastomosis of bowel to bowel was a rarity. After clinical introduction of the Murphy button, there was an explosion of interest for its use in gastrointestinal surgery and its application in that area enjoyed wide success in all parts of the world. Murphy also developed an oblong model for gastroenterostomy. Sir Berkeley Moynihan of Leeds praised the development of the button as the "most exquisite surgical implement ever invented."

Murphy's button was commonly used until about 1935, and sporadic use in the gastrointestinal tract continued well into the 1940s. John L. Keeley reported (9) using the oblong-type button for gastroenterostomy in a poor-risk patient at Charity Hospital in New Orleans in 1940 at the advice of a seasoned attending surgeon. In 1943 while on duty in the U.S. Navy at Pearl Harbor, Morris Friedell of Chicago noticed a Murphy button on a shelf in the operating room. Some time later, a seaman was admitted with a transection of the jejunum at the ligament of Treitz and he used the button to accomplish quickly a difficult union in a very sick patient (6).

Although the button was originally intended for bypassing the gallbladder and was then adapted for gastrointestinal anastomosis, it was also used in other ways. In 1918, H. P. Jack utilized the Murphy button for suprapubic drainage of the urinary bladder (8). In the 1940s, H. H. LeVeen modified a Murphy button for vascular anastomosis (10). He utilized Teflon for the device and altered it so as to evert rather than invert the edge. In 1943, L. Miscall (Bellevue Hospital) utilized the button for resection of carcinomas of the lower third of the esophagus (11). He emphasized that the particular advantage of the button is the provision of a tight, nonleaking anastomosis. As late as 1986, Prioton et al. reported using it for "portal disconnection" of the esophagus in cirrhosis patients with bleeding varices (14).

More recently yet, in 1990, two reports have appeared describing the use of a soluble "Murphy button" for gastrointestinal anastomosis, which is said to have advantages over the stapling techniques currently in use (1; 3).

The Murphy button may represent the first application of a temporary prosthesis within the human body. The principle of this button is
the basis of present-day stapling instruments.

MECHANICAL BOWEL OBSTRUCTION

Significant controversies existed in the early 1900s regarding the ad-
visability of performing surgical procedures on patients who suffered
from "ileus." It was commonly noted that surgical mortality rates
were twice those of patients treated nonoperatively, and some physicians wondered if all patients with intestinal obstruction should be
treated conservatively.

Murphy contended that observations favoring nonoperative approaches were biased to include cases of ileus occasioned by nonsur-
gical diseases. Because the most sophisticated laboratory tests available were the white blood cell count and urinalysis, Murphy relied
heavily on the history and physical examination to elucidate conditions requiring operative intervention.

Murphy used a schema to differentiate ileus on an adynamic, or
reflex, basis from that of mechanical origin. First, concurrent illnesses
such as pneumonia, lues, or lead poisoning were to be ruled out. Then
the diagnosis of mechanical obstruction was considered if colicky
pain associated with tympany or borborygmi was present. Ausculta-
tion of bowel sounds was of paramount importance in the serial eval-
uations of potential surgical conditions. If present, feculent breath or
emesis clinched the diagnosis and mandated surgery.

Murphy wrote:

> In the diagnosis of internal strangulation, no matter from what
> cause, we have exactly the same symptoms as in strangulated
> hernia, except the physical signs are different. The symptoms of
> internal strangulation are as follows: Pain in the abdomen which
> comes on suddenly, gradually increasing in intensity for the first
> half hour, followed by nausea and vomiting, and inability to
> produce bowel movement. . . . Peristalsis is very greatly in-
> creased and is most pronounced in the neighborhood of the ob-
> struction. This increase in peristalsis continues until peritonitis
> sets in. . . . Opiates paralyze peristalsis for hours and therefore
> should never be given in acute intestinal lesions as they obscure
> the symptoms and signs of the pathologic process. (JBM 39)

The ideal operative exploration was done through a vertical incision with attention to delineate the status of the terminal ileum.
"These cases [of intestinal obstruction] should be operated on at the

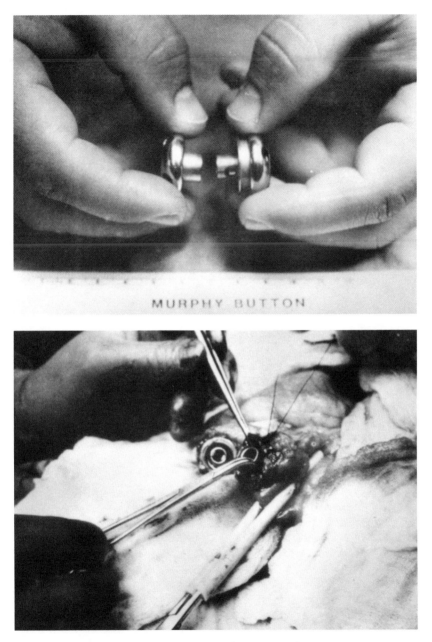

MURPHY BUTTON

Fig. 3.1. The Murphy button and its use for intestinal anastomosis.

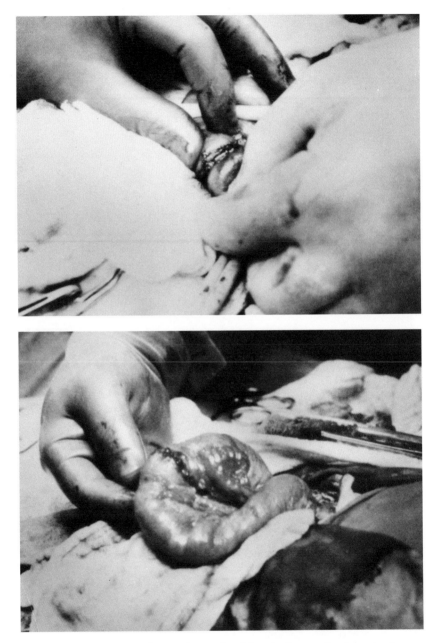

Fig. 3.2. Continuation of procedure using Murphy button for intestinal anastomosis.

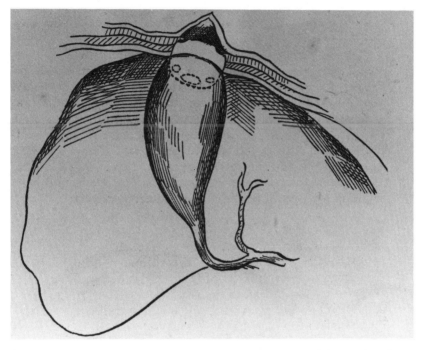

Fig. 3.3. The button used to bring the gallbladder to the abdominal wall.

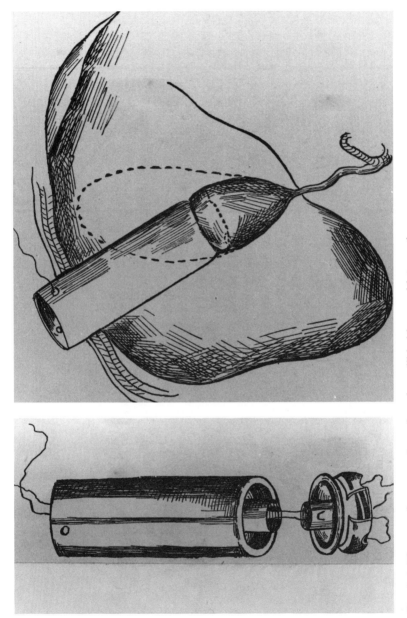

Fig. 3.4. The use of an extention when the gallbladder wouldn't reach.

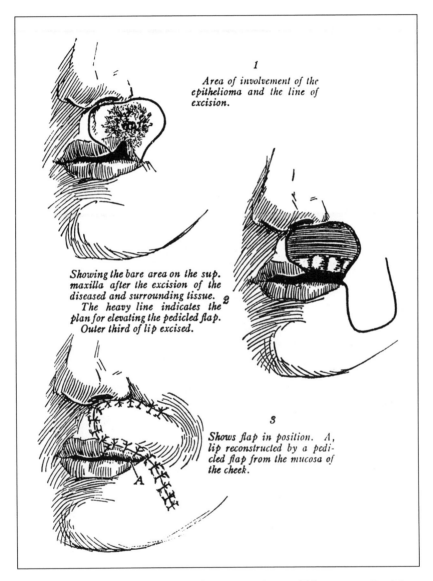

1

Area of involvement of the epithelioma and the line of excision.

Showing the bare area on the sup. maxilla after the excision of the diseased and surrounding tissue.
The heavy line indicates the plan for elevating the pedicled flap. Outer third of lip excised.

2

3

Shows flap in position. A, lip reconstructed by a pedicled flap from the mucosa of the cheek.

Fig. 3.5. Epithelioma of the upper lip starting in an old lupus scar. Excision. Plastic closure of the defect with formation of a new vermilion border to the lip by bringing down a small flap of buccal mucosa.

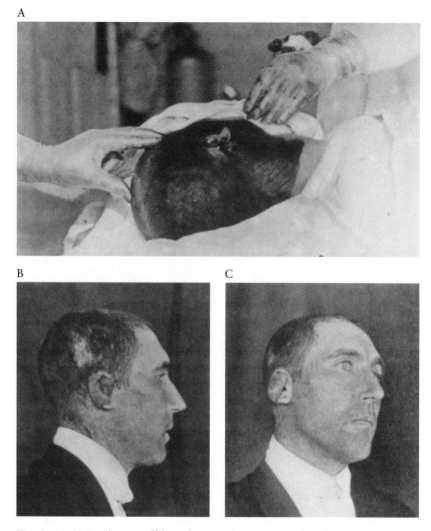

A

B

C

Fig. 3.6. (A) Ear bitten off by a horse. Photograph taken just before operation. All of the ear except the tragus and antitragus bitten off. (B) Lateral view, six weeks after operation. (C) Anterior view, six weeks after operation. The plastic flaps are visible in these photos. There is still some swelling of the tissues.

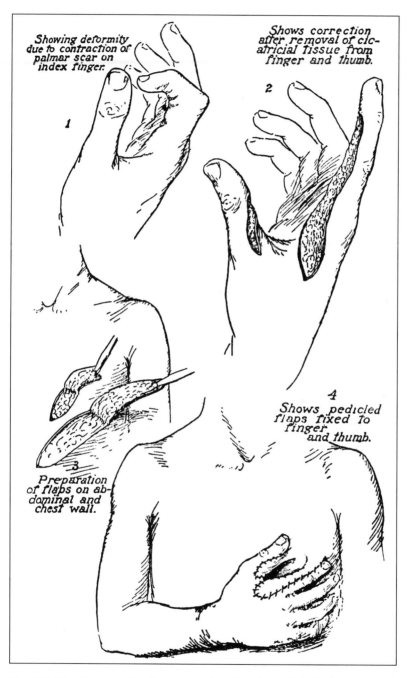

Fig. 3.7. Plastic operation for contracting cicatrices of the index finger.

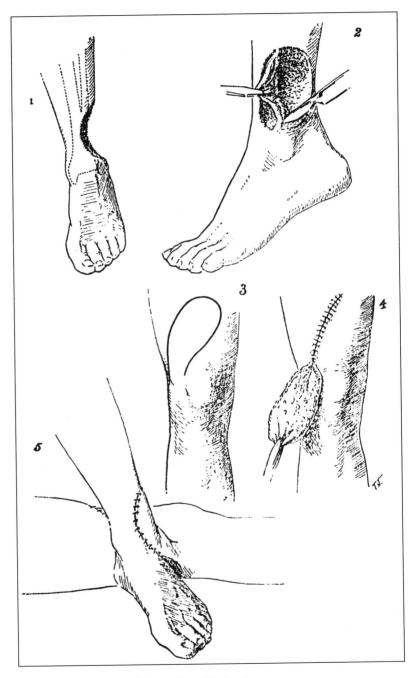

Fig. 3.8. A pedicle graft for a deep friction burn.

A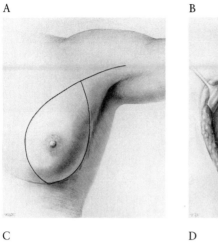

B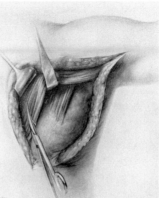

C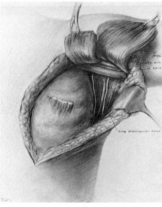

D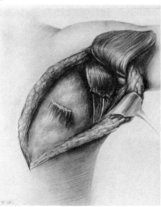

E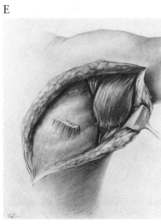

Fig. 3.9. Murphy's operation for cancer of the breast: (*A*) The incision. (*B*) The axillary dissection. (*C*) The pectorals have been separated from the chest wall. (*D*) The pectoralis minor turned into the axilla. (*E*) The pectoralis major turned in over the pectoralis minor.

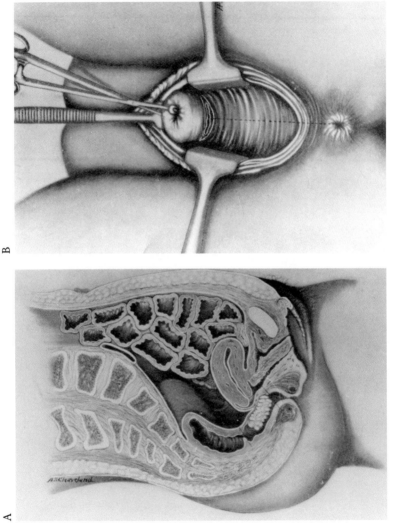

A

B

Fig. 3.10. Murphy's operation for a low rectal cancer (continued in figs. 3.11 and 3.12): (*A*) The location of the cancer. (*B*) Incising the posterior vagina.

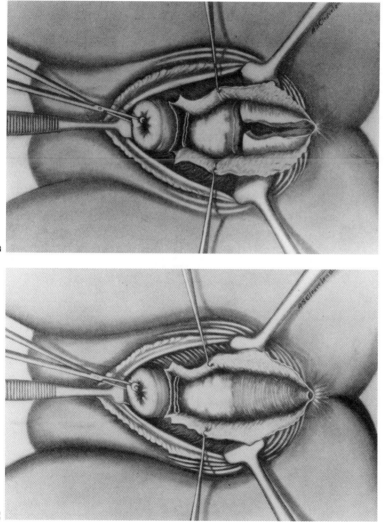

Fig. 3.11. (A) The rectum exposed. (B) The rectum opened and the bowel transected below the cancer.

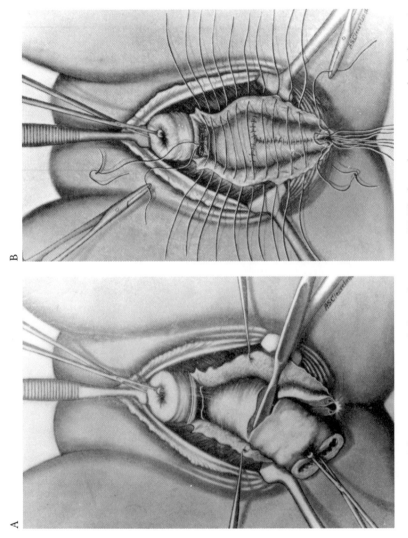

Fig. 3.12. (A) The rectum transected above the cancer. (B) The bowel reconstructed and the vagina about to be closed.

earliest possible moment before there is time for perforations, peri-intestinal adhesions, intra-abdominal abscesses or acute intestinal collapse, a condition from which the patient rarely ever rallies. Delay in operating for intestinal obstruction is more fatal than delay in any other abdominal lesion, except acute gastrointestinal perforations into the free peritoneal cavity" (JBM 111).

Non-edematous bowel allowed safe proximal exploration. Murphy emphasized the obvious need for care in handling obstructed bowel and the dangers of fecal spill in the peritoneal cavity:

> If the ascending colon be contracted you know the obstruction is above the ileocecal valve. Never allow the intestines to come out on the abdomen before you make the diagnosis. There may be pathologic conditions that compel you to do so, but not for diagnosis. . . . Just as soon as you find a contracted part you know you are below the obstruction. . . . If you run in the opposite direction . . . you come to the point of the obstruction. You can now liberate the obstruction, and you must do that without making traction on that part. I wish to warn you particularly. The tendency is to pull just a little more. The tissues have become friable, and you are liable if you make traction to tear the bowel and have the feces escape into the belly. (JBM 52)

The risks of ischemia and perforation from distension prompted Murphy to advocate decompressive enterotomy before closing. His mortality rates from operative interference were far better than those from the nonoperative treatment of "ileus," and his basic tenets still remain unchallenged.

SUPPURATIVE PERITONITIS

One century ago, survivors from suppurative peritonitis were rare and reportable. Most commonly, patients with this morbid entity suffered from appendicitis or from perforated peptic ulcers. Murphy elaborated factors influencing outcomes for those with suppurative peritonitis. In doing so he utilized contemporary thoughts about pathology and microbiology. He fashioned a cornerstone for critical care resuscitation by advocating more physiologic fluid resuscitation than was practiced at the time.

Evaluating the approach, he said:

> In discussing this very interesting subject, I would be ashamed to present such an appalling record were it not for the redeeming feature shown in the very gratifying results of the last thirty

cases. If we compare the first thirty cases operated on with the last thirty, we find as follows:

First series of 30 = 26 deaths; 4 recoveries.

Last series of 30 = 10 deaths; 20 recoveries.

To what is this striking difference due? There are two factors: (1) Improved technic; (2) earlier interference. (JBM 100)

Specifically, Murphy listed these risk factors in peritonitis (JBM 71):

a) The type of infection. If it be a virulent streptococcus type, with little pus formation, the peritoneum is rapidly denuded of the epithelial covering and becomes a "blistered surface," through which absorption rapidly takes place. Death in these cases is caused by the large quantity of the products of infection rapidly absorbed. If the poison be diluted or the pressure under which the infected products are retained be reduced the patient may pass over the critical period to a convalescence. If it be a staphylococcus or colon bacillus infection, the denudation is slower, the danger of immediate overpowering of the patient by the absorbed toxins is diminished and the fatal termination is postponed often to 4 to 6 days, until such time as the fibrinous exudate covering the peritoneum is exfoliated, taking with it the peritoneal endothelia. A rapid and fatal absorption may ensue.

b) The period of time that elapses between infection and the time of operation. In the past the diagnosis of perforation was based on a combination of symptoms included under the term collapse, which was believed to occur a few hours after the perforation took place. At present the diagnosis of acute infectious perforative peritonitis is based on the symptoms of pain, nausea and vomiting, localized tenderness, circumscribed flatness on piano percussion, elevation of temperature and hyperleucocytosis, in the order mentioned. With these symptoms many of the patients give a history of diseased conditions which predispose to perforative peritonitis. The operation should, therefore, be performed as soon as these symptoms are manifest. If it be postponed until the patient is in collapse the case will terminate fatally. If it be performed, however, in the early stage, the "peritoneal shingles" or endothelia will be found intact, thus preventing absorption. When these natural barriers to absorption are destroyed, as is the case when operation is delayed, a fatal outcome can not be obviated.

c) The tension under which the products of infection are retained in the peritoneal cavity. The mere presence of pus in this situation does not necessarily mean absorption of the infective products. The greater the pressure under which the pus is held in these acute conditions the more rapid the absorption. This is true, not only in the peritoneal cavity, but also in suppurations in the cellular tissue in any part of the body. Remove the pressure and there is an almost immediate cessation of absorption, as is shown by the sudden subsidence of the symptoms of infection after draining an abscess . . . not withstanding that pus remains in the cavity after it has been opened. The reduction of pressure is one of the basic principles in the treatment in cases of general suppurative peritonitis.

d) The diffusion of the infective material through the peritoneal cavity. It is well known that when this diffusion takes place in the upper half of the peritoneal cavity the danger is enormously increased, because absorption from this part is much more rapid than from the lower or pelvic portion. On this basis all patients were kept in the semi-sitting position, at an angle of thirty-five degrees . . . to allow the pus to settle into the pelvis where it could be carried off by the drainage tubes.

e) The administration of antitoxins and other substances to antidote or dilute the immediate depressing effects of the poisons absorbed from the peritoneum. Antistreptococcus serum and unguentum Crede were administered to our patients, on the conviction that they contributed to this result to some degree. Saline transfusions were given to some patients for the same purpose, as well as to increase the arterial tension when low.

f) The length of time the patient is kept under the anesthetic and the extent of manipulation of the intestines and other tissues to which the patient is subjected during the operation. The patients were not killed on the table. I believe a large number of lives are sacrificed in operations for general peritonitis by excessive manipulation of the infected tissues and by sponging and irrigation of the peritoneal cavity. If the patient becomes severely depressed, collapsed or shocked on the table, it is practically certain that death will ensue. . . . It is my belief that sufficient time can be saved by working under general anesthesia to more than compensate for the dangers attending its use.

Therefore it was Murphy's attitude that if the surgeon could intervene in situations that featured organisms of relatively low virulence (colon bacilli rather than streptococci), contained in relatively small areas (one quadrant of the abdomen rather than diffusely spread), recoveries could be anticipated if operative manipulations could be minimized.

Murphy argued against vigorous peritoneal toilet when operating for localized suppurative processes; he advocated an aggressive attitude toward surgical correction of perforated viscus or the common acute suppurative entities of appendicitis and cholecystitis in order to prevent generalized peritonitis; he recognized the tremendous absorptive capacity of the peritoneum and the dangers of toxemia; he advocated a "2 pint salt" resuscitation postoperatively via proctoclysis. By these tenets he produced six survivors from suppurative peritonitis in six months during 1902 (JBM 103).

Murphy assessed his method, writing:

> If I have added anything, it is in pointing out the importance of time in treating these cases, closing the hole, and not doing too much handling, drainage, and blood washing by proctoclysis. I did my work as carefully in the abdomen up to the time I made my previous report on the other cases in 1902 as I do now, but the patient died. Now they do not die. I believe this is not due to a change in the virulence or type of infection; these are the same practically as they always have been, and always will be, when the infection comes from the intestinal tract. No, the change in results is due to the timely intervention and type of treatment. (JBM 100)

Typhoid perforation will be discussed in Chapter 10.

THE MURPHY DRIP

By 1900 it was well established that fluid could be absorbed from the rectum and that this was an effective way to hydrate patients unable to take fluids by mouth. It was a treatment very popular with Murphy and he used it extensively in the treatment of peritonitis (JBM 103; *SC* 134). He published his method, utilizing drawings and photographs (JBM 108; *SC* 616), and for many years surgeons used the "Murphy drip."

Murphy outlined the method in this way:

> The apparatus in its simplest form consists of a fountain syringe or can with a large rubber tube attached, terminating in a vaginal hard rubber or glass douche tip flexed at an obtuse angle

two inches from its tip, having numerous openings in its bulbed end. The tip should be inserted into the rectum so that the angle fits closely to the sphincter, and the tube may then be bound firmly to the thigh with adhesive strips so that it may not be expelled. The bag or can is suspended from the foot of the bed so that its base is six inches above the level of the patient's buttocks. Once the irrigating apparatus is thus placed, it need not be disturbed for several days, unless to increase or decrease the speed of influx.

He continued, "The solution, consisting of a dram each of sodium chlorid and calcium chlorid to the pint of water, is now placed in the reservoir." (It was kept warm by various means, including a heating tube of Murphy's design that could be plugged into the electric light fixture.) The average amount given to an adult was "eighteen pints in twenty-four hours; that is, a pint and a half every two hours. The proctoclysis is usually continued for three days; rarely as long as five or six."

Proctoclysis remained a form of hydration well into the twentieth century, even after subcutaneous and intravenous routes became more acceptable, and more often than not it was referred to as the Murphy Drip.

MISCELLANY

There are many other areas of general surgery in which Murphy was quite active without making any special contributions. Most of these records appear in the *Surgical Clinics* but a few appear in his journal articles as well. To illustrate the range of his talents we review this material in outline form.

Trauma
Gunshot wounds of the abdomen (JBM 3):
  1. All should be explored;
  2. Make the incision through the wound of entry;
  3. Have a systematic plan for exploration;
  4. Always check the retroperitoneum;
  5. Close any bowel meticulously with two layers of catgut;
  6. Wash out the peritoneal cavity with boric acid solution;
  7. Use drains as indicated.
Trauma to the genito-urinary tract is covered in Chapter 9.

Head and Neck

Plastic:

1. Excision of an epithelioma of the nose with full thickness graft from the arm (*SC* 12; 35).

2. Repair of harelip and/or cleft palate (*SC* 39, p. 310; *SC* 595).

3. Excision of an epithelioma of the upper lip (in an old lupus scar) with a pedicle graft from the cheek (*SC* 337) (fig. 3.5).

4. Reconstruction of the nose with a pedicle flap from the arm (*SC* 365).

5. Bone graft for saddle nose (*SC* 366; 424).

6. Skin graft for contracted cicatrix of neck in burn scar (*SC* 559, p. 807).

7. Excision of leukoplakia with mucosal pedicle grafting (*SC* 421; 422; 423).

8. Reconstruction in stages for fracture of the malar bone with bone grafting, paraffin injection, and fascia lata grafting (*SC* 528).

9. Wiring together of the maxilla and mandible for gunshot fracture (*SC* 563).

10. Reconstruction of an ear bitten off by a horse (*SC* 139) (fig. 3.6).

11. Revisions of scars and contractures (*SC* 397; 432; 499) (fig. 3.7).

12. Pedicle skin grafting of a friction burn of the ankle (*SC* 353) (fig. 3.8).

13. Reconstruction of a badly lacerated thumb (*SC* 328).

Thyroid:

1. Excision of a cystic goiter (*SC* 44).

2. Excision of exophthalmic goiter (*SC* 73; 599).

3. Excision of a cystadenoma (*SC* 137).

4. Excision of a solid adenoma (*SC* 227).

5. Superior accessory thyroids (JBM 89).

6. Strumectomy for toxic goiter (*SC* 598).

Carcinoma:

1. Excision of carcinoma of the lip with partial lymphadenectomy and plastic reconstruction (*SC* 64; 367; 368; 560).

2. Excision of a sarcoma of the malar bone including the orbital surface (*SC* 361).

3. Excision of a malignant epulis of the mandible and a suprahyoid neck dissection (*SC* 362).

4. Enucleation of a parotid tumor (*SC* 364; 526).

5. Radical excision of carcinoma of tongue and neck through a neck incision (SC 396; 562).

6. Excision of the maxilla for malignancy of the antrum (SC 425; 565).

Miscellaneous:
1. Debridement of osteomyelitis of maxillary antrum (SC 369).
2. Excision of thyroglossal sinus (SC 426).

Breast

Carcinoma:
When doing radical mastectomy Murphy did not remove the pectoral muscles because they were seldom involved by the tumor, but he did take the fascia and the axillary lymphatics, carefully preserving the nerves. He developed a flap from the major pectoral, or occasionally from the latissimus or subscapularis muscle, to fill the empty axilla (fig. 3.9). A drainage tube was placed through a stab wound in the lower flap. He dressed the patient with the arm abducted 90 degrees in an airplane splint for ten days.

Stomach and Duodenum

Gastroenterostomy (done by button 75 percent and suture 25 percent):
1. For duodenal or gastric ulcer. In doing these operations, he sometimes mobilized the ligamentum teres and brought it tightly around the pylorus to force the stomach to empty through the new opening.
2. For congenital pyloric stenosis in a female (SC 112). Gastroduodenostomy: For perforating duodenal ulcer after its excision (SC 311).

Small and Large Bowel

1. Tuberculosis was resected only if the peritoneum was free of disease, otherwise the obstructed bowel was bypassed, even by colostomy if necessary, or the patient was treated with rest and tuberculin injections.
2. Malignant tumors and various granulomas were resected rather conservatively and continuity was reestablished by suture or button anastomosis.
3. Several abdominal fecal fistulas were explored and treated with resections or bypass procedures.
4. Hirschsprung's disease was treated by forceful dilatation per

rectum (*SC* 183).

5. Carcinoma of the rectum was usually treated by first establishing a colostomy and doing a second-stage posterior resection. On five occasions, he did a transvaginal resection and end-to-end anastomosis (JBM 58) (figs. 3.10 through 3.12).

6. Operations were done for imperforate anus with rectovaginal fistula (*SC* 295) and with perineal fistula (*SC* 359).

7. A presacral dermoid was resected (*SC* 518).

8. Rectal prolapse was treated by retroperitonealizing the rectum transabdominally and amputating the redundant prolapse by cautery from below (*SC* 33).

Miscellaneous

1. Inguinal hernias done by the Andrew's technic, illustrated in *SC* 175.

2. Ventral hernias done by an imbrication technic, illustrated in *SC* 513.

3. Two patients with mesenteric fibromas (JBM 59; 93).

REFERENCES

1. Bubrick, M. P., et al., "Prospective, randomized trial of the biofragmentable anastomosis ring," *American Journal of Surgery* 161 (1991): 136–43.

2. Clapsattle, H., *The Doctors Mayo* (Minneapolis: University of Minnesota Press, 1941), 310.

3. Dyess, D. L., P. W. Curreri, and J. J. Ferrara, "A new technique for sutureless intestinal anastomosis," *American Surgeon* 56 (1990): 71–75.

4. Ellis, H., *Famous Operations* (Media, Pa.: Harwal, 1926), 28.

5. Fitz, R. H., "Perforating inflammation of the veriform appendix," *Transactions of the Association of American Physicians* 1 (1886): 107; *American Journal of Medical Sciences* 92 (1886): 321–46.

6. Friedell, M. T., personal communication, 1989.

7. Herrick, J. B., *Memories of Eighty Years* (Chicago: University of Chicago Press, 1949), 73.

8. Jack, H. P., "Suprapubic drainage of the urinary bladder," *JAMA* 70 (1918): 1225.

9. Keeley, J. L., "Remembering the Murphy Button," *Mercy Hospital Medical Center Journal* 5 (1988): 22.

10. LeVeen, H. H., "Nonsuture method for vascular anastomosis utilizing the Murphy Button," *Archives of Surgery* 58 (1949): 504–10.

11. Miscall, L., and B. B. Clark, "The Murphy Button in esophagogastrostomy," *Surgery* 14 (1945): 83–87.

12. Morton, T. G, "Inflammation of the vermiform appendix, its results,

diagnosis and treatment," *Maryland Medical Journal* 22 (1889): 404, 484; ibid., 23 (1890): 8.

13. Musgrove, W. W., "Dr. John B. Murphy," *Manitoba Medical Association Review* 17 (1937): 201–6.

14. Prioton, J. B., et al., "Long-term results after portal disconnection of the esophagus using an anastomotic button," *Surg. Gynecol. Obstet.* 163 (1986): 126.

4

GYNECOLOGY

Robert L. Schmitz

As was true for most surgeons at the time, Murphy's surgery included a wide variety of gynecologic procedures. They made up about ten percent of his volume. Many of his journal articles and his reports in the *Surgical Clinics* deal with gynecological problems and describe his personal operative techniques, several of them unique.

UTERUS

Murphy preferred the vaginal approach to hysterectomy, even for uterine cancer, because of its lower mortality rate. In his early technic, he left clamps on the broad ligaments and held them in place by vaginal packing (*SC* 436; JBM 46). The clamps were removed in forty-eight to seventy-two hours and the packing in two weeks. With this technic he reported a mortality of only 2.5 percent, remarkable for the time. Later he stated that he seldom used the clamp method anymore, preferring to suture the broad ligaments since it was more comfortable for the patient (*SC* 436, p. 1147).

While discussing vaginal hysterectomy he remarked, "I have seen four hours and fifteen minutes consumed in performing a simple hysterectomy for uncomplicated carcinoma of the cervix—an operation that should be performed in from ten to twenty minutes. I have seen it done in seven minutes" (JBM 46, p. 202).

In spite of his preference for the vaginal route, Murphy did do hysterectomy from above if it was indicated, for example, in the case of large fibroids. He noted, "The method of abdominal hysterectomy which we employ is original with us, so far as we know" (*SC* 115, p. 183). It consisted of approaching the uterus from behind to better expose the ureters and to better control the uterine and ovarian vessels, which were separately ligated. The uterus was amputated supracervically and the "abraded surfaces" were carefully reperitonealized (fig. 4.1).

When hysterectomy was done for cervical cancer he said, "I prefer the vaginal . . . route for the extirpation of the uterus for malignant disease, though recently the abdominal route has been urged in preference because it permits of the removal of the retro-peritoneal carcinomatous glands. This is only a theoretical advantage and is more than counter-balanced by the increased mortality of the abdominal route" (JBM 46, p. 211). He denigrated the Wertheim operation again in a second paper (SC 36, p. 278).

Retroversion he considered to cause backache and pelvic discomfort and to be a major factor in infertility and sterility. He wrote,

> In the cure of retroversion there are two plans of procedure. If you have a retroversion with descensus of the uterus . . . then you have to do some operation which either fixes the uterus to the anterior abdominal wall or you have to take the uterus out. . . . In an ordinary retroversion in a nullipara without an enlargement of the uterus and without pelvic inflammation . . . the operation as we have done it here for eight years is folding the round ligament over the dome of the uterus, suturing it there. This shortens the round ligament and tips the uterus forward. (SC 79; SC 560, p. 831)

He cautioned that ventral fixation for retroversion should never be employed in a woman capable of becoming pregnant.

The *Surgical Clinics* cite several approaches to procedentia: pessaries, suspension, ventral fixation, hysterectomy, and translocation of the uterus into the anterior abdominal wall. This last procedure he did with the fundus intact or split in two. This operation is described in *SC* 150: "If we see the case in the early stage, we do a ventral implantation; that is, we implant the fundus of the uterus between the divided aponeuroses of the abdominal rectus muscles. [The broad ligaments were first separated.] If it is a superlative degree case . . . split it anteroposteriorly into two halves, take out the mucous membrane entirely . . . lay the two parts of the uterus, serous surface forward, on the rectus sheaths, like the two wings of a bat, and suture them with catgut" (fig. 4.2).

Most dysmenorrhea he thought to be of the "obstructive" type, i.e., stenosis of the external os. For this he did the Pozzi operation: After dilating the cervix, he said, "I take out a V-shaped piece of the muscularis from the cervix. That permits of approximation of the outer and inner surfaces of the mucosa. . . . The stitches are put in so as to catch the columnar epithelial cells on the inner side, and the squamous epithelial cells on the outer side, bringing those into accurate apposition, so that there will be no possibility of a transverse healing" (*SC* 79).

What we term functional uterine bleeding Murphy referred to as essential hemorrhage of the uterus (*SC* 115). He also used the term "fibrosis uteri" (*SC* 115, p. 193), which is probably what we call adenomyosis today. In general, abnormal bleeding was classified as essential hemorrhage, incomplete abortion, inflammatory, or from fibroids. He often used uterine packing for heavy bleeding in spite of the fact that he describes a complication produced by another surgeon's packing which suggests the toxic shock syndrome as we know it (*SC* 87, p. 807). He was cautious about curettage late in incomplete abortion because he feared septicemia.

In a patient he explored to uncover an explanation for her amenorrhea, he discovered a total nonfusion of the Mullerian ducts. The individual halves of the uterus had been drawn into the inguinal canals by the round ligaments. After reducing them, he sewed the two halves together to prevent this recurring but did nothing more. In his discussion, he gave an interesting review of the embryology of the uterus (*SC* 548).

ECTOPIC PREGNANCY

He diagnosed ectopic pregnancy mainly by a careful history and clinical evaluation (*SC* 521). While there was a test for pregnancy available at the time, the Abderhalden test, it was complicated and lengthy and was no match for the present-day pregnancy tests.

The test was based on chorionic protein being present in the mother's bloodstream from the sixth week of gestation until fifteen days after delivery in quantity enough to be detected. The chorionic protein produces antibodies that can be detected by colorimetric technic after exposing them through dialysis to placental tissue. The test was neither specific nor sensitive enough, it was very complicated to prepare and to perform, and it usually took a full day to get the result. Even so, Murphy used the test frequently as an adjunct to diagnosis and discussed it at length in two places (*SC* 222; 299). Later he said, "We are trying to check up all our uterine fibroid cases with the Abderhalden test, in order to get at its practical value in these cases" (*SC* 338, p. 298). No reference appears in regard to the results.

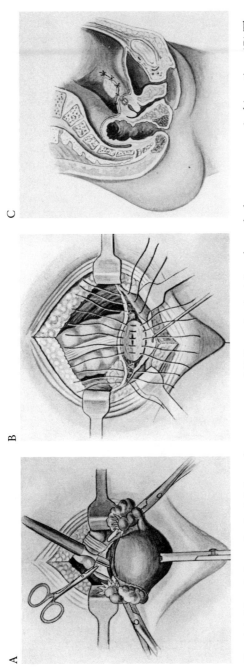

Fig. 4.1. Murphy's method of doing a hysterectomy: (A) Posterior incision through the corporocervical junction. (B) The cervical sutures and broad ligament in place. (C) The cervical sutures tied and the abraded surface covered with peritoneum.

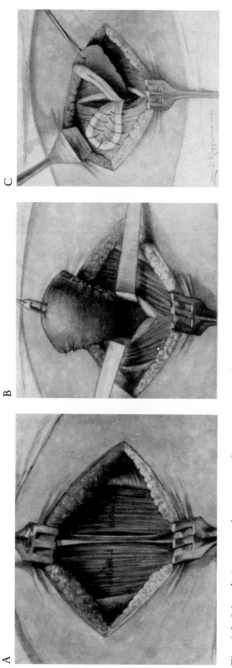

Fig. 4.2. Murphy's unusual operation for severe procedentia: (A) The incision. (B) The uterus drawn up after dividing the broad ligaments. (C) The uterus split and being tacked down over the rectus muscles. Drawings appeared originally in Bryant and Buck, *American Practice of Surgery.*

APPENDICITIS IN PREGNANCY

Not surprisingly, the problem of appendicitis in pregnancy was of great interest to Murphy. "There is a colossal mortality percentage when one does not operate, and only a slightly lower percentage when one does operate, except in the cases that are operated within the first few hours of the attack, before the disease has become a constitutional infection" (*SC* 299). He continued, "If one operates for appendicitis in pregnancy in the first six or eight hours of the attack, as one can in all these cases, when its importance is grasped by the physician and properly impressed on the patient, the mortality should be very slight."

OVARY

Murphy emphasized the degree of torsion in relation to symptomatology in ovarian tumors, in pedunculated fibroids, and in volvulus of the G-I tract. He made a differentiation between two-fifths rotation without vascular compromise and three-fifths with first venous and then arterial occlusion. He had occasion to demonstrate several cases of 240 degree twists of ovarian tumors or pedunculated fibroids which induced thrombosis in the blood supply and precipitated an acute abdomen (*SC* 13; 252).

In view of the still unsettled classification of ovarian neoplasms, it is not surprising that Murphy's references to them are confusing. There was a tendency for him to consider tumors to be benign cysts only to have them recur as evident cancers, and he spoke more commonly of ovarian sarcomas than carcinomas.

Many patients with recurrent ovarian tumors were explored in an effort to palliate them. After such an operation at which he was able to resect a large recurrent mass of "cystosarcoma," he said, "This patient will be put on large doses of arsenic, hypodermically; that occasionally retards growths of this type, and occasionally retards them in a very striking manner" (*SC* 78). And again after a similar operation, "We shall give her large doses of sodium cacodylate—five, six, seven, eight, or ten-grain doses at a single injection. In the cases in which we have given this drug our results have been excellent. You can see usually a pronounced diminution in the size of the tumor. . . . We do not recommend this drug as a cure, and we are not writing about it yet. For some of these cases we have used 606. . . . We intend using the sodium cacodylate intravenously as soon as we can get someone to do the experimental work to prove its safety" (*SC* 252, p. 609).

PELVIC INFECTIONS

During an operation being done by Dr. John Golden for salpingitis, Murphy gave the audience a discourse on pelvic infections with a detailed scheme of classification (*SC* 87). He was aware of the very high mortality that was associated with tubovarian abscess and felt bilateral salpingectomy was usually indicated; the ovaries were spared if at all possible (*SC* 108). However, if the patient was youthful, he would even attempt to leave the tubes intact if there seemed to be any chance of patency (*SC* 522).

Pelvic tuberculosis was a common complication of the disease and was frequently seen in tuberculosis hospitals. Murphy wrote one of his comprehensive review papers on "Tuberculosis of the Female Genitalia and Peritoneum"; its length required three issues of the *American Journal of Obstetrics and Diseases of Women and Children* for publication (JBM 65). His usual treatment stressed conservatism and involved bilateral salpingectomy with careful burying of the tubal stumps, since he had seen two cases of fistulization to the small intestine. Following the surgery, the patients were put on tuberculin therapy, usually for at least six months.

MISCELLANEOUS

Several other gynecologic reports are of interest:

1. A fibroma of the vaginal wall large enough to interfere with pregnancy (JBM 40; 42).

2. An abdominal pregnancy removed thirteen years later (JBM 79).

3. Five rectal cancers removed through the vagina (JBM 58, covered in Chapter 3).

4. An attempt to repair a fecal fistula to the vagina following an attempted abortion (*SC* 189).

5. A uterine fibroid complicating pregnancy excised and the defect repaired without disturbing the fetus (JBM 40).

5

NEUROSURGERY

Michael J. Jerva and Robert L. Schmitz

Murphy's papers contain several articles in neurosurgical areas as well as a sizable monograph on surgery of the spinal cord and peripheral nerves (JBM 99). In addition, there are frequent case reports in the *Surgical Clinics*.

In many of the presentations of neurosurgical cases before his visitors in the operating theater, Murphy asked the neurologist Charles Louis Mix to describe the neurological findings and together they made dramatic predictions of what would be found at surgery.

At the conclusion of an operation for "phlegmon of the spinal cord" Murphy expressed some rather startling ideas:

> It does not matter how this case terminates: there is still the great feeling of satisfaction of knowing that, by operating, we gave the patient a chance for her life. Not only do I appreciate Dr. Mix's assistance in establishing the clinical diagnosis, but I am also gratified that he was on hand to see the living pathology, which adds so much positiveness to the medical phase; I have frequently expressed the feeling that every surgeon should associate himself with the best internist available and, per contra, that every internist should associate himself with the best surgeon available. There should be no specialists in medicine: they should be "universalists" by cooperative team work. (*SC* 478)

PERIPHERAL NERVES

His earliest writings concerning peripheral nerves dealt with trigeminal neuralgia (JBM 37; 38). He tried surgery on the Gasserian ganglion, first extracranially and then intracranially (JBM 110). Of the latter operation he says, "We have done altogether some 16 or 18 Gasserian ganglion removals, that is, complete removals, securing in all cases in which we have been able to get reports permanent relief" (SC 75). After cutting the nerve roots, he filled the foramen from inside with a Murphy plug, a coal-tar-paraffin preparation, to prevent regeneration, which was a problem in most cases. In 1904, however, he reported that out of twelve intracranial operations, he had four deaths and felt that was too high for a disease that did not threaten life (JBM 84). Therefore, he reported, "We have resorted to the easier and safer procedure of extradural exposure of the nerve" (SC 75). He also tried osmic acid injections and enthusiastically reported a series of fourteen patients in 1904 (JBM 84). But here again the benefit was mostly short lived, so the problem was never solved for him.

Peripheral nerve repair intrigued Murphy and he experimented endlessly in his laboratory, trying different technics including cable grafts. He has recorded in detail how repair can be effected (JBM 97; 99; 113; SC 4; 14) (fig. 5.1).

While the neuron theory (regeneration is dependent on the neurilemma) was not generally accepted, he was confident that it was valid. He felt it was incumbent upon the surgeon to attempt peripheral nerve repair even though paralysis had been present for years; he believed that "no matter how long a nerve has been divided, if you recontact the ends without the intervention of connective tissue, you will have regeneration in the distal axonal portions. We had one case where the nerve was reunited 26 years after its division and function was restored" (SC 42, p. 346). He reiterates this attitude in another article and points out that even atrophic muscles can regain tone and strength (JBM 97).

Decompression of tardy ulnar palsy from scarring could be very rewarding and he would operate even after years had gone by; he cautioned that it may take as long as eighteen months for any regeneration to become evident (JBM 97; SC 231; 232; 400).

Operations on peripheral nerves by him included three brachial plexus repairs. He dissected out the fasicles and reanastomosed those that were injured (fig. 5.2); his description of the anatomy is superb (SC 42; 320). He demonstrated two years later the excellent outcome of one of these patients who had had end-to-end anastomosis of the seventh and eighth cervical-segments and the median, musculocutaneous, and musculospiral nerves. All functions were now intact (fig. 5.3.). As Murphy said, "The result speaks for itself" (SC 124).

Anastomosis, transplantation, and transection were performed on a variety of peripheral nerves including spinofacial, ulnar, musculo-spiral, median, external popliteal, brachial plexus, and cauda equina, always using the principles that were enumerated in his writings and summarized in his monograph on neurological surgery (JBM 99).

The problem of phantom limb bothered him but he did not devise a satisfactory solution. He was willing to explore the stump for a neuroma and when he found one he tried to avoid a recurrence "by dividing the nerve in such a manner that it will heal . . . by means of the proliferation of glial tissue in the large axons. Glial repair is established thus. The nerve end is not cut squarely across, but it is cut across transversely for one-half of its diameter at a point three-fourths of an inch from its end; this cut half is split vertically downward to the end of the nerve, and is then removed. . . . The nerve end is folded back upon the nerve and stitched to the heel of the bayonet-shaped nerve-end" (JBM 44; SC 418) (fig. 5.4).

In one patient he blamed the phantom pain on ascending neuritis rather than a neuroma and transected the cauda equina on the side of the amputation (SC 230). A few weeks after the operation the pain had recurred. Six months later, Murphy reexplored this patient's cord and resevered the cauda. At the time, faradic stimulation showed no transmission of motor function to the leg stump; nevertheless the patient was totally continent of stool and urine (SC 261). Following this second procedure, "pain was frequent and referred to different portions of the amputated extremity, but it is now gradually abating."

SPINAL CORD

For trauma to the spinal cord, Murphy emphasized early decompression. His case reports include lesions of the cord and cauda equina (SC 111; 217). Even in old injuries he was willing to explore with the hope of excising organized hematomas or thickened dura (SC 113; 217; 455; 456). In posterior spinal dislocation with compressive myelopathy, he recommended open reduction.

He realized that paralysis of motion had a different prognosis from "paralysis of sensation" and that in concussion of the spine (now called the central or anterior cord syndrome) there could be complete recovery after decompression (SC 61). A complete transverse paralysis from injury would never recover cord function but a victim who still had some sensation or motor function below the level of the injury could improve, and decompression would help (JBM 98). "Once the true cord is cut, it never regenerates, no matter how accurately it is approximated" (SC 61).

During laminectomy, he wrote, "it simplifies the operative procedure to remove the laminae and the spinous processes, and one can remove them readily in the majority of cases and without detriment to the patient or traumatizing the cord" (*SC* 113). In a patient with tuberculosis of the thoracic spine with marked kyphosis and lateral deviation and symptoms of cord compression, he removed the spinous processes and laminae of the fourth, fifth, and sixth dorsal vertebra. In another patient with a benign bony tumor that he chose not to excise, he removed five spinous processes, C8, T1–4, and four laminae (*SC* 385). No bone grafting was done in these cases.

Whenever he wanted to avoid sewing the dura back together for fear of recompressing a swollen cord, he used the erector spinae muscle. He explained:

> We will take this erector spinae muscle with its smooth fascia from the side, and throw the muscle forward in between the edges of the dura, turning it over with its smooth fascia toward the cord and suturing it to the edges of the dura so as to get a 3/4-inch expansion of the lumen of the dural canal. This insures a permanent release of the cord from transverse dural compression [fig. 5.5]. This is a new procedure as far as we are able to find out, and was original with us, we believe, though it is dangerous to claim originality in anything since the excavations in Asia Minor have disillusioned us on so many supposed modern originalities.

He reported using this technic several times (*SC* 217; 354; 386; 387).

While operating to remove a bullet lodged in the upper dorsal vertebral canal, he criticized earlier care elsewhere:

> In this case a double mistake was made of probing for the bullet and catheterizing the patient. Never catheterize when the trauma involves the spinal cord. Why? Because the greatest mortality in injuries to the spinal cord comes from bed-sores and infections of the urinary bladder and the kidneys. . . . Just let the bladder fill with urine. After two or three days, if the patient is a woman, massage the sphincter vesicae through the vagina; if the patient is a man, massage the sphincter through the rectum. Finally, there is relaxation of the sphincter and the urine begins to flow. (*SC* 157)

He also attacked spinal-cord tumors for cure and palliation (*SC* 168; 171), even operating on recurrent lesions (*SC* 76; 173), and in some instances was able to remove completely benign and malignant tumors.

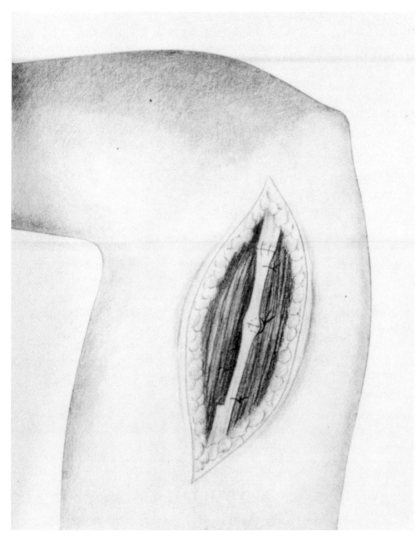

Fig. 5.1. The median nerve stretched and ends sutured together.

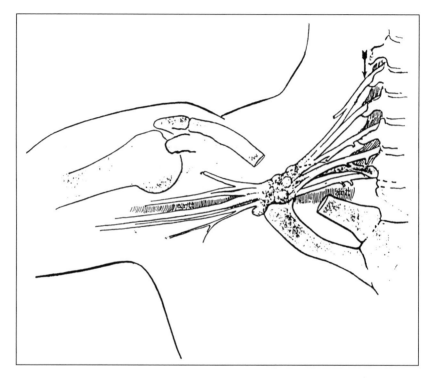

Fig. 5.2. The pathological situation in one of the brachial plexus injuries treated by Murphy. He dissected out the fasicles and reanastomosed them with good result.

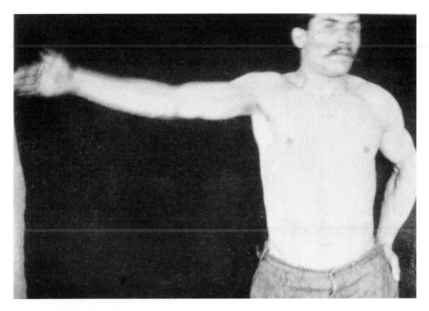

Fig. 5.3. An excellent functional result two years after a brachial plexus repair by Murphy.

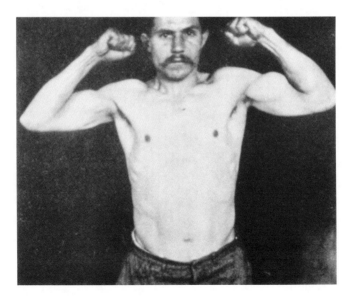

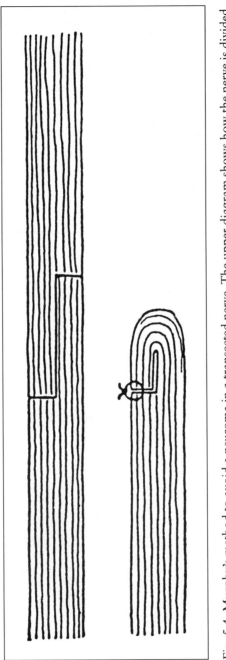

Fig. 5.4. Murphy's method to avoid a neuroma in a transected nerve. The upper diagram shows how the nerve is divided. The lower diagram shows how the end of the stump is turned up to contact with the upper cut end and effect axonal contacting.

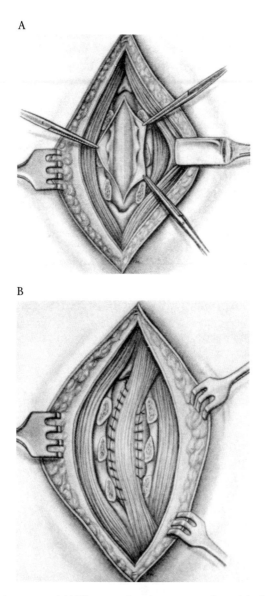

Fig. 5.5. Laminectomy. (A) The cura has been opened, and is drawn to both sides to expose the cord, which is flattened out by the cicatricial tissue running across it. (This schematic drawing does not show the scar tissue.) (B) A strip of the erector spinae muscle has been drawn over and sutured into the gap in the dura to prevent subsequent pressure on the cord by cicatricial tissue, a procedure that was original with Murphy.

The *Surgical Clinics* include operations for spina bifida and meningocele. One of the patients was only one month of age (*SC* 125). Murphy tried injecting Morton's fluid, a combination of iodine, potassium iodide, and glycerine, without success and concluded that "excision of the sac seems to be the radical and most desirable procedure" (*SC* 125). The articles include photographs, roentgenograms (skiagrams), and drawings.

In the last volume of the *Surgical Clinics* (*SC* 455) there is a "Bibliography of cases of injury, disease, and neoplasms of the vertebral column or spinal cord previously published in the clinics." The list is included here to demonstrate the extent of Murphy's experience. The page numbers follow the month and year of publication of the *Surgical Clinics*.

1. Injury:
   Traumatic cervical spondylitis. August 1915, 713.
   Impacted fracture of the body of first lumbar vertebra. April 1913, 275.
   Concussion of spine with impacted fracture of vertebra. August 1912, 545.
   Compression of cord from traumatic angulation of first lumbar vertebra. February 1914, 161.
   Fracture-luxation of spine at twelfth thoracic vertebra. December 1914, 1077.
   Fracture-luxation of second lumbar vertebra with compression of cauda equina. See following case, p. 59.
   Luxation of spine at second lumbar vertebra. Open reduction. February 1915, 109.
   Bullet in lumbar spine. August 1913, 601.
2. Disease:
   Cicatricial constriction of cord. August 1915, 741.
   Typhoid spine. June 1912, 429; August 1915, 745.
   Pott's disease: Talk by Dr. Fred H. Albee. June 1913, 455.
   Tuberculoma of spinal column with compression of cord. December 1913, 1011.
   Tuberculous granulomas of vertebrae. August 1915, 731.
   Subcutaneous abscess following tuberculosis of the spine. December 1913, 1027.
   Tuberculosis of the thoracic spine with compression of the cord. February 1915, 67.
3. Neoplasms:
   Intradural cystic tumor. April 1915, 368.
   Bony tumor of spinal canal. August 1915, 719.

Endothelioma of spinal cord. October 1912, 695; August 1913, 733. (Contains table of tumors of cord.)
Myeloma of cord. August 1913, 709.
Intrathoracic sarcoma starting from vertebral column. October 1914, 883.
4. Congenital deformity:
Spina bifida; meningocele. April 1913, 265.

BRAIN

Murphy saw many patients with trauma to the head. He taught that "a patient who receives a blow on the head, whether there is evidence of fracture or not, who is not rendered unconscious, does not get epileptic convulsions; while a patient who receives a severe blow on the head and becomes unconscious, whether there is evidence of fracture or not, later in life very frequently gets epilepsy" (*SC* 42, p. 340).

Post-traumatic epilepsy or personality disorders he treated by excising the scarred and thickened dura or residual hemorrhagic cysts in the area of involvement. Following the excision he placed a thin layer of paraffin over the brain to prevent adhesions to the brain. Murphy remarked, "The question comes up in all these cases as to why we have the epileptic convulsions. Are they due to the irritation of the dura, or are they due to irritation of the brain? That has not been definitely settled, but it is my conviction, from clinical observation and from some experiments made years ago, that it is the irritation of the dura that causes the convulsions" (*SC* 62).

Through burr holes Murphy evacuated extradural and subdural hemorrhage and clipped the bleeding vessel; however, he made an alternative suggestion, especially if craniotomy was not immediately feasible: "All you need to do when you feel that the patient is going into a state of coma on account of rupture of the middle meningeal artery is to make a little incision under cocain anesthesia, salt solution, or sterile water analgesia, cut down on his external carotid, and throw a ligature around it" (*SC* 50). Elsewhere he noted, "After one has tied off the external carotid artery, whatever clots have already accumulated outside or inside the dura will necessarily remain there. But they are not liable to do any further harm than has already been inflicted, and they can be removed by craniotomy at a later period, if necessary" (*SC* 370). Compressed fractures were explored and debrided (*SC* 372).

Murphy was willing to try to decompress posterior fossa tumors (*SC* 128; 174) and in one instance he partially resected a glioma of the cerebellum. He did not report the total excision of any brain lesions, however. It was in the postoperative management of brain tumors that Murphy evaluated a pulmotor. (See Chapter 7.)

These operations were done by Murphy when neurosurgery was just beginning to be established as a specialty by Sir Victor Horsley (1857–1916) in London and by Harvey Cushing (1869–1936), "the Father of Neurosurgery," in the United States. In contrast to Murphy, they regularly excised brain tumors (some two thousand for Cushing), but they did little work with pheripheral nerves or spinal-cord trauma. Cushing did operate for trigeminal neuralgia and devised a sensory root interruption rather than the total extirpation Murphy used. Cushing also decompressed the spinal cord for tumors. To counteract cerebrospinal fluid leak he did a tight fascial closure in contrast to Murphy's muscular closure. Murphy's neurosurgery was done in addition to much other surgical work while Horsley and Cushing stayed exclusively in their field.

6

ORTHOPEDICS

Robert L. Schmitz and Gerald F. Loftus

Murphy had orthopedic patients throughout his career, but the volume of such cases increased greatly beginning in 1910. He became particularly involved with arthritis, arthroplasty, and bone grafting. As always, his approach to these problems included preliminary experimental work.

One of his orthopedic articles is actually a sizable monograph in which he reviewed most of his work (JBM 120). He divided the text into three main areas—bones, joints, and tendons—an easy division to use for the present chapter.

Murphy's operative technique for orthopedic operations was somewhat different from that for other procedures. Lane technic was used; everything was done with instruments; the hands never touched the skin or the wound.

The skin was painted with tincture of iodine. The deep fascia was closed with phosphor-bronze wire, the superficial soft tissues with chromicized catgut, and the skin with interrupted silkworm-gut retention sutures and horsehair interrupted in the edges. Drainage was rarely used.

After the iodine had been removed from the skin, the field of operation was freely dusted with bismuth subiodide powder and sealed with gauze soaked in collodion. A large pad of gauze saturated with 5 percent phenol was placed over the entire field and then a sterile dressing and spica bandage were placed over all.

Murphy cautioned repeatedly about circular casts or tight roller bandages whenever there might be swelling, for fear of ischemic contractures such as Volkmann's. Whenever circular casts were used, one or two Gigli wires were incorporated and as soon as the cast was dry, it was split along its anterior margin.

BONES

One of Murphy's interests was bone grafting. He did much animal work to establish his principles, and the "laws" he composed are still valid and worth quoting in detail:

1. The periosteum fully detached from bone and (1) transplanted into a fatty or muscle-tissue bed in the same individual, if he is young, may produce a lasting bone deposit; (2) transplanted into another individual or animal of the same species and under the same conditions, it rarely, if ever, produces a permanent bone deposit; (3) transplanted into another species it never produces a permanent bone deposit.

2. Periosteal strips elevated at one end from the bone and attached at the other, if turned out into muscle or fat, reproduce regularly bone on their under surface for a greater portion of their entire length.

3. Transplanted into other individuals or animals of the same species and contacting at one end with exposed or freshened bone it rarely produces permanent bone, even for a small extent at its basal attachment, and never produces bone for its full length.

4. Bone with its periosteum transplanted into muscle, fat, etc., in the same individual, and free from bony contact, practically always dies and is absorbed, except in the case of very young children or infants. Transplanted into another species it is always absorbed.

5. Bone transplanted without the periosteum into muscle or cellular tissue always dies and is ultimately absorbed.

6. Bone with or without periosteum transplanted in the same individual and contacted with other living osteogenetic bone at one or both of the ends of the transplanted fragment always becomes united to the living fragments and acts as a scaffolding for the reproduction of new bone of the same size and shape as the transplanted fragment if asepsis is attained. This new bone increases to such size as is necessary to give the support required by Nature in the extremity in which it has been placed. It will scaffold the production of new bone even into the joint when it is surrounded by capsule, and tuberosities are produced in about the regular location, as in the normal conformation.

7. The transplanted fragment, no matter how large or how small, is always ultimately absorbed. The role it plays is to give mechanical support to the capillaries and blood-vessels with their living osteogenetic cells, as they advance from the living

bone at both ends of the transplanted fragment into the haversian canals, canaliculi and lacunae of the transplant. New lamellae are deposited around the new capillaries and these lamellae fit into and adjust themselves in the graft, so that the bony union is actually formed and mechanical support given long before the transplant is entirely absorbed and replaced by new bone. Ultimately all of the transplant disappears as new lamellae are firmed by the osteoblasts, and the graft lamellae are removed by osteoclasts.

This conclusion is based on my observations and on analysis of the microphotographs and pathologic specimens, clinical and experimental, presented by others. . . .

8. The graft increases in size on the surface as bone increases in size histologically, i.e., by deposits beneath its newly-formed periosteum.

9. The muscles should be fixed or directed to the graft in the same relation as the normal anatomic fixation, if muscular control is expected after the graft has become united, and the musculotendinous attachments should be accurately sutured to the graft at the point of desired union, either with catgut or phosphor-bronze wire.

10. Bone covered at end by cartilage and on the sides by periosteum, such as the phalangeal bones, even when contacting with living bone denuded of periosteum, dies, and is wholly absorbed. When the graft is covered with periosteum at the point of contact with the living bone, the haversian vessels do not penetrate the fibrous periosteum of the transplant, and regeneration fails. If the periosteum of the graft is split into shreds, then regeneration through it may take place.

11. Periosteum attached to the transplanted portion, if the graft is taken from young individuals, has a plus osteogenetic influence; in the middle-aged it is neutral; in those of advanced years it plays a minus role and, in fact, it is detrimental.

While these theories may finally be found defective in some of their details, they represent my observations in the experimental and clinical work I have carried on. (JBM 120)

Murphy used bone grafting frequently in five areas: ununited fractures; replacement of bone lost through infection; replacement of bone removed in the treatment of tumors; defects of bone development, whether congenital or acquired; and stabilization of the spine after fracture/luxation or tuberculosis.

The donor site for the graft was usually the crest of the patient's opposite tibia. He had his own retractor-guide for obtaining the bone (fig. 6.1). When grafting ununited fractures he placed the graft intramedullarly across the fracture site after using his reamer to make space (fig. 6.1). In all these maneuvers his bone skid was an invaluable tool (figs. 6.1 and 6.2).

While Murphy was adept at closed reduction for fresh fractures, he did not hesitate to use open reduction when he thought a better result would be obtained nor to use foreign materials for fixation when indicated. But he warned against putting foreign materials into compound fractures.

When fractures involved the olecranon, the condyles of the humerus or femur, or the malleoli of the ankle, he liked to make a small nick in the skin and drive an eight or ten penny nail through the fragment into the shaft of the respective bone (fig. 6.3). Various other materials used as implants and fixaters included an ivory peg for a phalangeal fracture, ordinary wood screws across fracture lines, phospho-bronze wire for muscle and tendon suturing (fig. 6.16), and an occasional Lane plate in an open reduction.

Sometimes he inserted magnesium ribbons at right angles to each other in the medullary canal across the juncture of bone ends to stabilize the union (fig. 6.3). The ribbons slowly decomposed causing the release of considerable quantities of hydrogen gas at the operative site, which accumulated beneath the skin and had to be aspirated from time to time.

Spinal fracture-luxations were approached by open operation with the objective of decompressing the cord (see Chapter 5). At times he might insert a bone graft for stabilization.

Open operations were often used to correct healed fractures with poor alignment and function. In these instances fixation with nails, screws, wire, or plates was more common than bone grafting since there was usually not the problem of nonunion (fig. 6.2).

For ununited fractures, Murphy also used open reduction with fixation, especially for nonunions of the neck of the femur. But he more frequently used bone grafting (figs. 6.1, 6.2, and 6.4).

When operating on the hip, he often detached the greater trochanter and reflected it superiorly with its attached muscles to more clearly expose the joint. The trochanter was reattached at the completion of the operation by nailing. This was true whether or not a graft was used.

If the lunate was dislocated without fracture, it was reduced; a fractured scaphoid was given a chance to heal; when a lunate or scaphoid fragment became aseptic it was removed; in an instance of an old dislocation of the capitate with necrosis, the entire bone was removed.

A fractured patella was wired together when feasible. If wiring was not feasible, he used a strip of quadriceps tendon that was still attached at its patellar end, passed it through the patellar tendon below the fracture, and fixed it upward under tension, thus locking the fractured pieces together. It was a method he had devised in 1904 in the treatment of tuberculosis of the patella.

When fractures entered joints, Murphy emphasized exact reduction and firm casting to preserve the joint as much as possible. In contrast, for fractures of the bone shaft, he recommended loose casting to allow some motion at the fracture site to promote healing.

The nonspecific varieties of osteomyelitis he treated by making multiple drill holes in the affected bones, removing sequestra and saucerizing cavities. After the disease burned itself out, if there was missing bone in an important location, he replaced it with a graft (fig. 6.5).

Typhoid and tuberculous osteomyelitis were treated in a similar manner, unroofing the abscesses, curetting the cavities, removing sequestra, and placing drains (fig. 6.6). Then for acid-fast disease the part was immobilized and tuberculin therapy was administered. He cautioned against placing any foreign materials in an actively infected area and yet he would graft the spine while active tuberculosis was still present.

Several operations for tuberculosis of the patella are described. If there was only a pocket of infection he recommended removing any sequestra, curetting the cavity and filling it with "our glycero-gelatine-formalin plug." If there was more involvement, the patella was removed, taking care not to enter the knee joint. After the removal of the bone, a pedicle of quadriceps tendon was turned down from above and sewn to the edge of the tendon left below from the extirpation of the patella.

Murphy thought that bone sarcoma was initiated by a single trauma that was not severe enough to produce a fracture. Murphy was reluctant to amputate for such bone tumors unless there was no alternative, and he locally excised several sarcomas (giant-cell, chondro, and spindle cell), even including the joint space, and inserted long bone grafts to establish usable extremities (fig. 6.7). When he thought that a lesser procedure would not do, however, he did not hesitate to do radical operations including major amputations, disarticulations, and even an interscapulothoracic quarterectomy for a recurrent osteosarcoma of the humerus.

Using an unusual procedure, he excised the entire scapula for osteosarcoma in a young woman, leaving the arm in place. He attached the capsule of the joint and the trapezius muscle to the acromion. She had a very usable extremity.

A patient who had been operated on for cancer of the breast four and one-half years before seemed to have a solitary metastasis to the head and neck of the femur. He excised the upper femur and in a second stage inserted a bone graft, hoping of get a functional limb. There was no follow-up.

A hemimandibulectomy was done for a giant-cell sarcoma in a ten-year-old girl; he replaced the missing bone with a previously prepared silver prosthesis (fig. 6.8) (JBM 120). In 1959, the *Chicago Tribune* reported that a California oral surgeon got the surprise of his life when a sixty-year-old woman with a fractured jaw handed him her X-ray. The break had occurred not through bone but through silver. When the patient was ten, Dr. J. B. Murphy had resected half her jaw and had replaced it with a custom-made silver implant, which had been working perfectly for over half a century (1).

He was interested in osteitis fibrosa cystica. He thought it resulted from trauma, often minor, followed by a low-grade infection. "These cases, we believe, are infections with absorption of bone, but an infection of a low type in which the products have a stimulating effect on the osteoclasts which absorb the bone, or an inhibiting effect on the osteoblasts" (SC 177, p. 804).

When a lesion interfered with the function of an extremity or joint, either of two approaches was used. Murphy might resect the involved portion of the extremity, including the head if it was involved, and replace it with a graft (fig. 6.9). Or he might simply unroof the lesion, curette out the diseased area, and lay in a bone graft (fig. 6.10). He even did the latter in a patient with the disease only in the phalanx of a finger.

Simple solitary cysts of bone were treated by curetting out the cavity and fracturing the shell of the cyst into the cavity for the purpose of obliterating the cavity by new bone formation.

Some insight into Murphy's ego is revealed in the following anecdote. A patient had a destructive lesion in the shaft of the femur; Murphy made a diagnosis of a granuloma. He exposed the tumor, unroofed it, curetted it thoroughly, and filled the cavity with Moorhof's bone wax under dry conditions. He said the mixture would solidify as the wax was absorbed and would be replaced with fibrous tissue or bone. The pathology report came back as mixed-cell sarcoma. In an editor's note Murphy said that "the pathologist's diagnosis did not confirm the clinical diagnosis of granuloma. The history and skia-

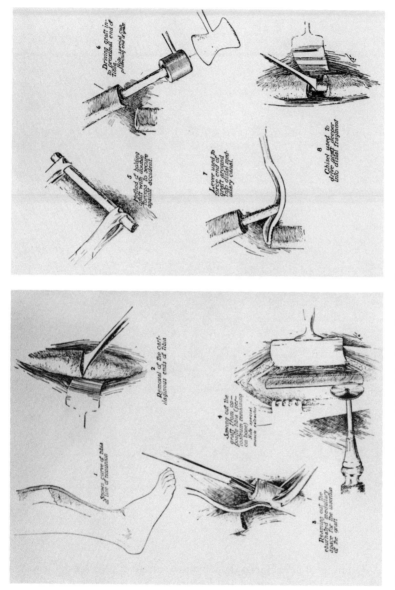

Fig. 6.1. A series of drawings, with original numbering, illustrating Murphy's method of bone transplantation for nonunion of the tibia. In drawing 2 the cartilaginous covering of the bone-ends was not clearly outlined by the artist.

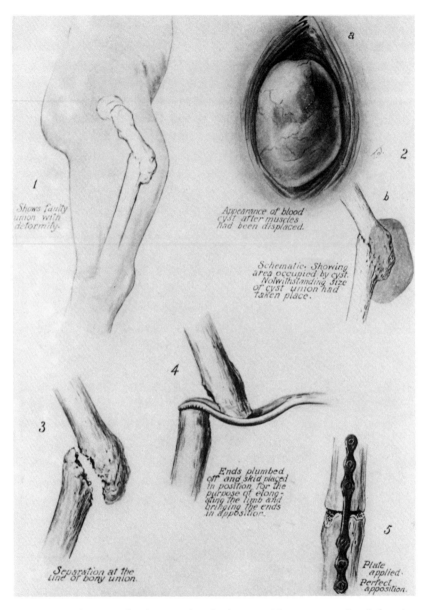

Fig. 6.2. Malunion of a fractured right femur with great angular deformity (anterior bowing). Open reduction and fixation with a Lane plate. Large cyst of hemorrhagic origin found at the fracture site.

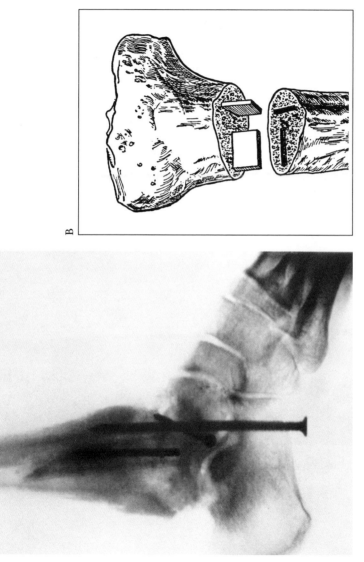

Fig. 6.3. (A) X-ray of case of Charcot ankle taken fifteen days after operation. (B) Method of using magnesium ribbon splints in bones. Two splints in position in upper fragment with slots in lower fragment, into which splints would fit when proper approximation was made, thus maintaining separation and desired elongation as well as normal position.

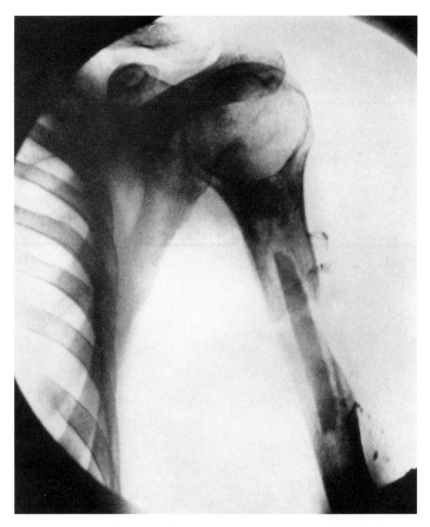
Fig. 6.4. Ununited fracture of humerus after operation, showing bone splint transplanted from tibia.

A   B

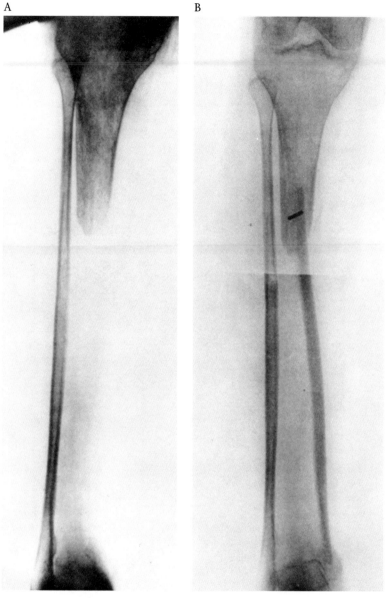

Fig. 6.5. (A) The X-ray of an osteomyelitic destruction of the femur. (B) The same patient six weeks after bone-grafting. The nail in the upper fragment prevents the graft from slipping. Murphy said that on the "skiagram" new bone could be seen forming along the graft ends.

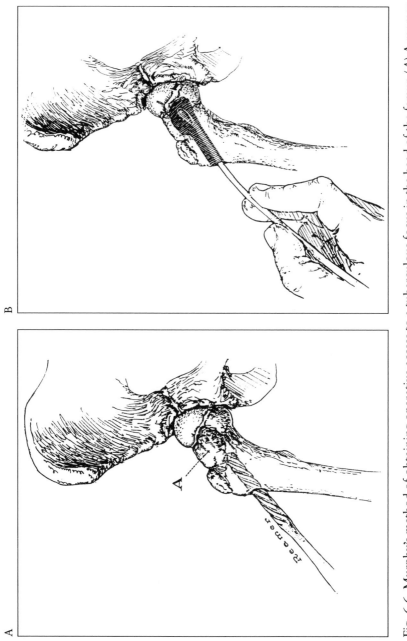

Fig. 6.6. Murphy's method of obtaining operative access to a tuberculous focus in the head of the femur. (A) A reamer was passed through the neck into the abscess. (B) The cavity is curetted. The resulting space was filled with iodoform. Thus the integrity of the femoral head was maintained in contrast to sacrificing it by resection.

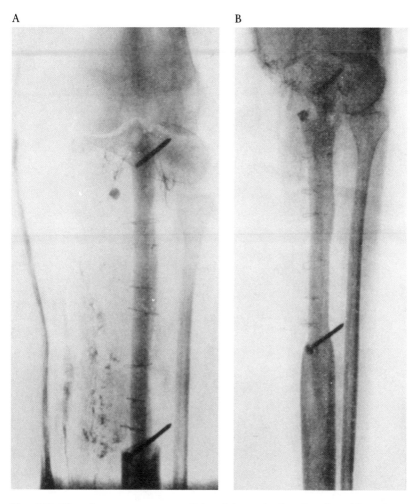

A   B

Fig. 6.7. Chondromyxosarcoma of the tibia excised and replaced by a long
bone graft. (A) X-ray taken through the cast a few days after the operation.
(B) X-ray taken five weeks after surgery. The graft has thickened and the
lower end shows bony union.

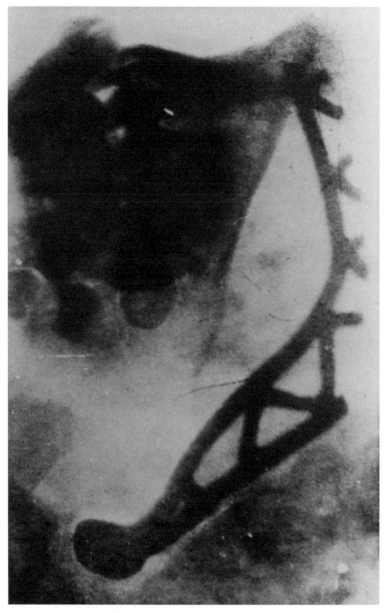

Fig. 6.8. Metal jaw in position following resection of right inferior maxilla for neoplasm.

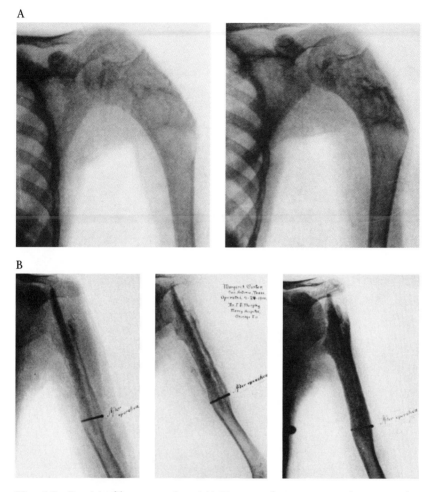

Fig. 6.9. Osteitis fibrosa cystica. (*A*) X-rays taken two months apart; the progress of the disease is seen from left to right. (*B*) X-rays taken ten weeks, sixteen weeks, and seven months after resection and bone grafting show the progressive reconstitution of the humerus around the graft.

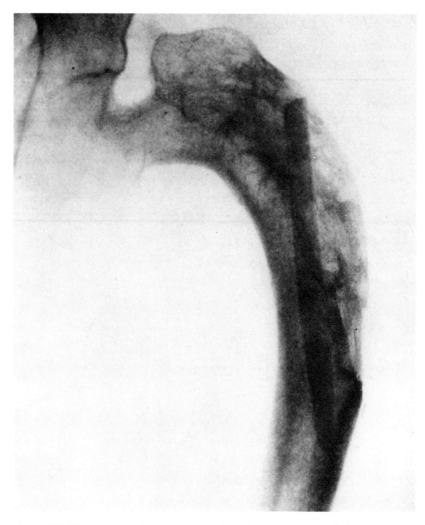

Fig. 6.10. X-ray made about seven weeks after an inlay graft for osteitis fibrosa cystica of the upper femur. New bone is forming around the transplant

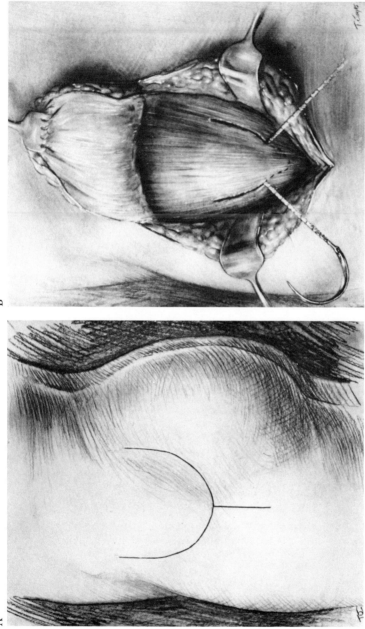

Fig. 6.11. The essential steps in arthroplasty of the hip by Murphy's fascia-and-fat flap method (continued in figs. 6.12 through 6.14). (A) The incision. (B) After the flap of skin, fat, and fascia lata are reflected upward, the chain saw is passed under the superior muscle group and the trochanter is detached and swung upward.

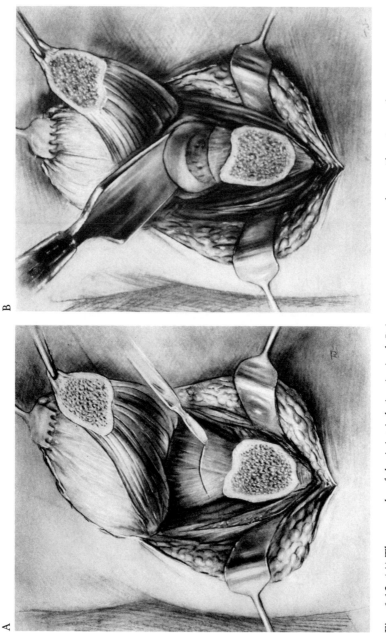

B

A

Fig. 6.12. (A) The capsule of the joint is being incised. It is not necessary to cut the pyriformis or obturator externus muscles. (B) A gouge that fits the normal curve of the head of the femur is driven between the head and the acetabulum to divide the ankylosis.

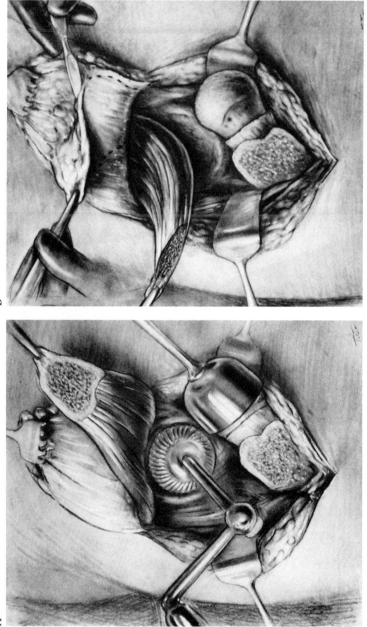

Fig. 6.13. (A) The head of the femur and the acetabular cavity are reshaped and smoothened using Murphy's end-mill and reamers. (B) A pedicle of fascia lata and fat is prepared from the reflected incisional flap to be interposed between the freshened femur and acetabulum.

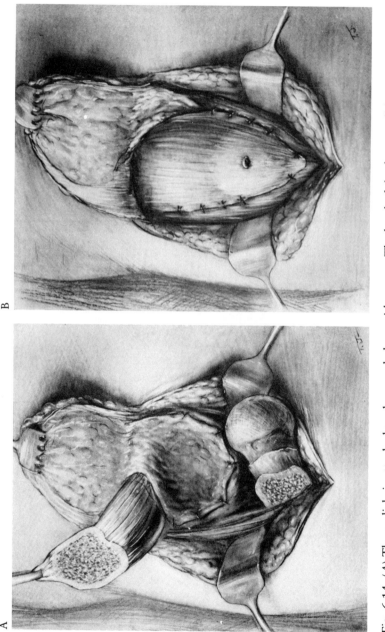

Fig. 6.14. (A) The pedicle is attached to the acetabulum with catgut. The head of the femur will be rotated onto it. (B) The muscle flap is reattached with a continuous suture of phosphor-bronze wire, and a nail is used to reattach the trochanter. The skin is closed with horse hair and silk-worm gut.

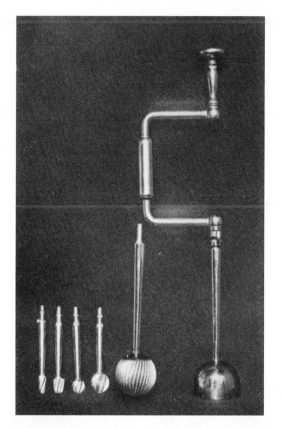

Fig. 6.15. Rongeur and burrs and neck conformer used by Murphy in arthroplasty of hip joint. These were apparently modified from Hudson's instruments.

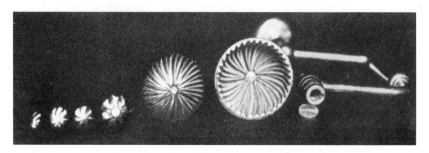

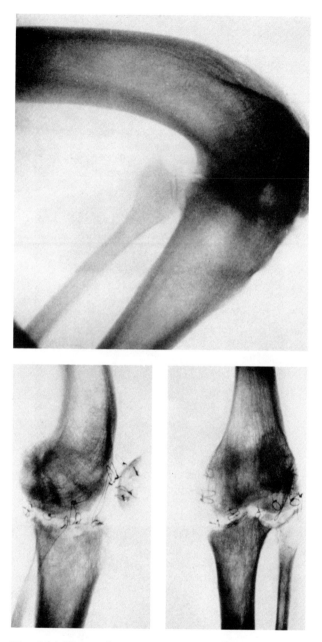

Fig. 6.16. X-rays showing ankylosis of the knee and the result after operation.

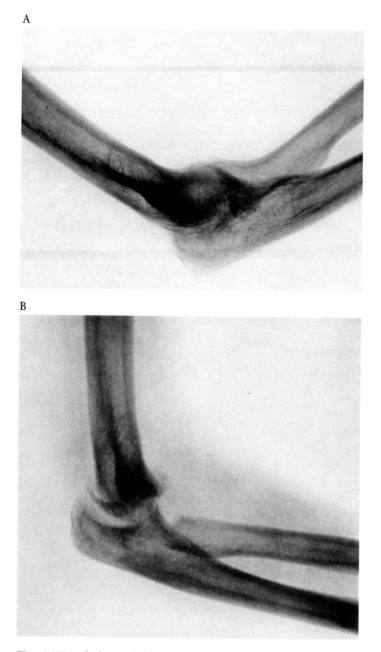

Fig. 6.17. Ankylosis of the elbow. (*A*) The preoperative X-ray. (*B*) The postoperative result.

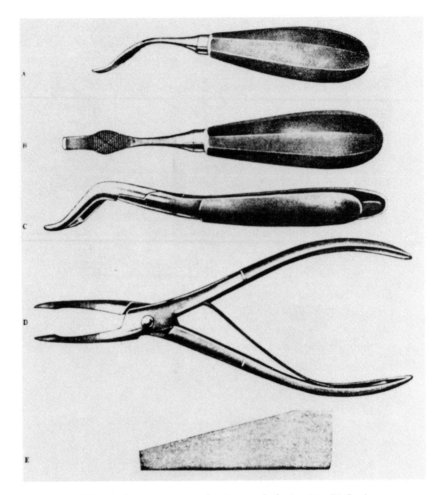

Fig. 6.18. Murphy's instruments for jaw ankylosis. (A, B) Periosteotome. (C, D) Bone-cutting forceps or nippers. (E) The interdental block made of wood.

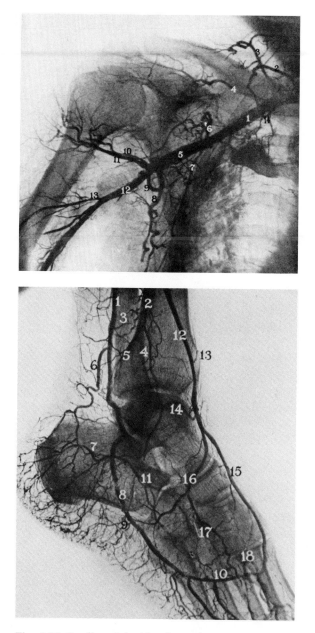

Fig. 6.19. Studies of the blood supply around joints to aid in flap design for arthroplasties.

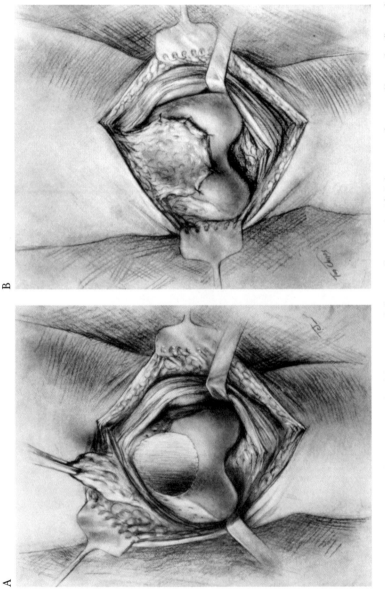

A

B

Fig. 6.20. Operation for congenital subluxation of the patella. (A) Artificial groove for patella and a flap of fascia-and-fat. (B) The flap is being interposed.

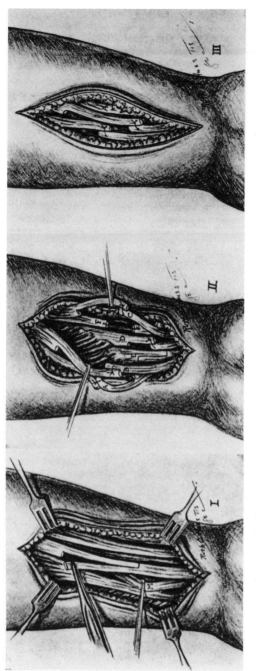

Fig. 6.21. Tenoplasty in the forearm. The tendons have been lengthened. Fat and fascia are sutured over the unions to prevent adhesions to the skin.

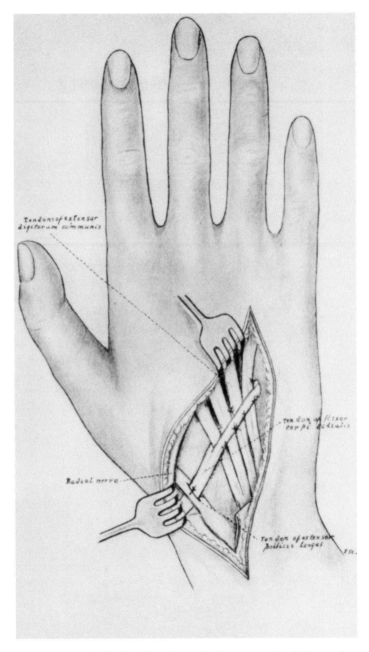

Fig. 6.22. Method of tacking the split flexor carpi radialis tendon to the front and rear of the extensor tendons of the digits.

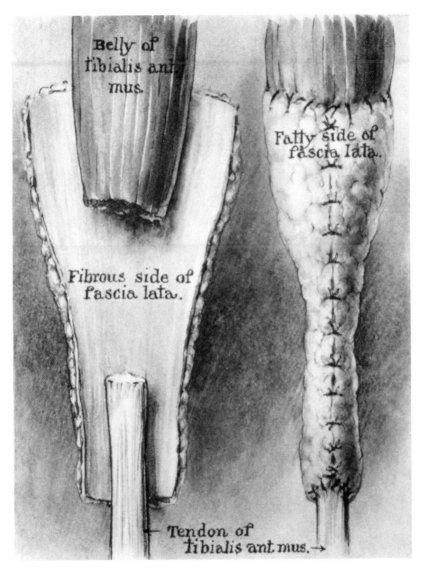

Fig. 6.23. Repair of tibialis anticus muscle.

gram confirmed the clinical diagnosis. The subsequent course of this case may determine which of these interpretations was correct."

Murphy did some interesting procedures to replace defects in bone. For patients with saddle nose deformity he made an incision along the side of the nose, cut a graft from the ulna, tibia, or fibula longer than necessary, and trimmed it after insertion. He made sure the graft was in contact with periosteum-free bone; a small incision at the tip of the nose might be made to help place the graft.

He attempted to use a phalanx from a patient with hyperdactyly for a nose graft, but failed to put the bone in contact with other bone or periosteum. After an initial good result, it slowly absorbed over the course of a year.

On another occasion he attached the hypothenar eminence of the hand to the nose, using the fifth metacarpal bone shaft as the graft. He held it there for two weeks and got a successful take even without bone contact because the graft had not been detached from living tissue. In a way, this operation heralded the multitissue pedicle transplants of today.

The defect in the chin of a man who had a shotgun injury was corrected with a tibial graft; various congenital deficiencies in long bones were corrected with bone grafts; cuneiform osteotomies of the tibiae were done for genu varum.

JOINTS

Murphy had a major interest in what he called metastatic arthritis. He wrote, "One of the reasons why the profession has been so tardy in recognizing the connection between the primary infections, as of the nose, pharynx, tonsils, skin, gall-bladder, typhoid ulcer or urethra, and the secondary arthritides, is that a long period of time elapses between the primary infection and the secondary arthritides in a large percentage of cases" (JBM 120, p. 40).

The primary infections were most commonly gonorrheal, influenzal, staphylococcal, streptococcal (scarlatinal), typhoid, or pneumonic. The joint localization was the result of "trauma or exposure, as wetting of the feet, playing in the snow, chilling in swimming, over or long-continued exertions" (JBM 120, p. 41).

Murphy said, "It is my conviction that every type of non-traumatic joint inflammation is a metastatic manifestation of a primary infection in some other portion of the body. It is my further conviction that there is no idiopathic rheumatic arthritis, any more than there is an idiopathic peritonitis" (JBM 120, p. 40).

Whenever a joint seemed to be at risk (from trauma, infection, arthritis), he liked to inject five to fifteen cc of a solution of 2 percent formalin in glycerin into it and apply Buck's extension. This solution needed to be prepared at least twenty-four hours in advance for the formalin to go into solution in the glycerin. He also used that solution a week or so before opening any joint. He felt that when the joint was opened there would be increased immunity against infection which could in turn produce ankylosis.

To Murphy, metastatic arthritis was a serious entity. He wrote, "It took nearly twenty years to have our 'early treatment of appendicitis' accepted. Let us hope the arthritides will not have to pay so frightful a toll before the treatment is accepted or disproved or supplanted" (*SC* 184, p. 861). Interest in these metastatic arthritides eventually led to extensive investigations of vaccine therapy, as detailed in Chapter 10.

In tuberculous arthritis—if the infection was healed—he occasionally did an arthroplasty, but when there was evidence of active infection, which was more commonly the case, he did an arthrodesis. In the knee joint this was the Murphy "concavoconvex" arthrodesis. It consisted of resecting the femoral articulation convexly and the tibial articulation concavely and fitting the resultant surfaces together. The leg was then casted until healing had occurred. In a young person, he might subsequently do an arthroplasty after healing had taken place because a movable joint was such an asset.

Neisserian arthritis was treated by injecting his solution of formalin in glycerin into the joint and applying Buck's extension.

Syphilitic joints were usually attacked with his standard arthroplasty. For one Pott's fracture in a Charcot ankle Murphy did an open reduction with nailing (fig. 6.3, left), but in another he did an arthrodesis.

When ankylosis was present, Murphy attacked it vigorously by arthroplasty. His principles were to excise all scar tissue so as to free up the joint and to interpose fascia, muscle, or mucous membrane to prevent recurrence. As always, these operations had been designed by appropriate experiments on dogs. In his 1991 book *Total Joint Replacement* William Petty says that Murphy "is considered the leader of his era in interposition arthroplasty" (2).

Murphy did his first arthroplasty on October 5, 1901, in a patient who had had gonorrheal arthritis and had ankylosis of both knees. He operated on both joints in stages, cleaning out all adhesions and interposing an attached pedicle of fascia lata in the joint proper and a smaller, similar pedicle behind the patella. The result was good, and hundreds more such procedures followed on the hip, knee, ankle, shoulder, elbow, wrist, and jaw.

The technique of arthroplasty on the hip was described in *Surgical*

Clinics 256 and is illustrated in figures 6.11 through 6.14. Murphy designed his own instruments for this operation, apparently modifications of those of Hudson (fig. 6.15).

Postoperatively the patient was placed in a Rainey travois splint which abducted both limbs, and twenty pounds of Buck's extension were applied to the affected leg. On the seventh to tenth day passive motion was begun. The splint was continued for three to four weeks. Then active motion was begun first on crutches and then unaided.

These same principles were used for other ankylosed joints with appropriate modifications. In the knee the patella was freed with scalpel and chisel. The patella and its ligament were retracted and the femur was separated from the tibia with scalpel and chisel. A pedicled flap of vastus externus or internus or lateral rectangular flaps from the inner and outer sides of the joint capsule were interposed between the femur and tibia behind the patella (*SC* 292) (fig. 6.16).

For the patella, after freeing that bone he occasionally split it and rotated the external half under the internal fragment to make a new articular surface. More frequently, he simply freed the patella from the femur and interposed nearby soft tissue (*SC* 208).

For ankylosis of the shoulder he had designed a technique on the cadaver but he had no opportunity to use it (*SC* 533).

In the elbow, after cleaning out the joint, an interposing flap was taken from the aponeurosis of the supinator longus and from the fascia and fat on the inner side of the joint (*SC* 293). After the operation, the elbow was immobilized at a right angle in a posterior and lateral plaster splint. Passive motion was begun on the fifth to seventh day and the splint removed permanently on the tenth day, when active motion was also begun (fig. 6.17).

In the wrist, the interposing flap was developed from the deep fascia and from the joint capsule (*SC* 307). In the jaw, usually a U-shaped flap of fascia and fat was turned down from the temporal muscle to interpose in the freshly cleaned joint (*SC* 253), but on two recorded occasions he used palatal mucous membrane (*JBM* 126). He would remove the coronoid process or maxillary condyle if necessary. Again, he designed his own instruments (fig. 6.18).

For an old fracture-dislocation of the metacarpalphalangeal joint of the middle finger, he excised a wedge from the involved metacarpal head, rotated the remaining fragment over the sawn base of the head, and thus formed a new articular surface.

In any of these joints, if there was not enough local tissue to use for interposition, as in patients who had already had multiple operations or who had had a destructive arthritis, Murphy took free grafts from the patient's fascia lata with good results.

Another area of investigation pursued by Murphy was the definition of the blood vessel pattern around joints to allow him to design better his various flaps for arthroplasty. Murphy had cadavers prepared in the Northwestern University Medical School Department of Anatomy. Professor Ranson injected the appropriate vessels with a red-lead emulsion. The preparations were then skiagrammed by Dr. George Hochrein, who did the radiographic work in Murphy's clinic. And finally, the various arteries were labeled by Sumner Koch, who was an assistant working in Ranson's laboratory at the time. Two illustrations testify to the excellence of this work (fig. 6.19). There are eight more in the collection (*SC* 155; 575).

The *Surgical Clinics* contain numerous reports in regard to trauma to joints. These can be summarized in the following list:

1. Torn or fractured semilunar cartilages were excised.

2. Hypertrophic villous synovitis was treated by synovectomy.

3. Acute bursitis was treated conservatively unless it became infected; infected bursae were drained.

4. For chronic bursitis the bursa was removed in toto. Such operations were reported for prepatellar, olecranon, trochanteric, and sub-Achilles bursae.

5. For congenital subluxation of the patella, he made a new bed for the patella in the front of the femur (fig. 6.20). In the acquired type, he did only tendon imbrication since there was already a good bed for the patella. By 1914 he had done forty-seven operations on the patella for subluxation.

6. For recurrent dislocation of the head of the humerus he tried capsulorrhaphy.

7. Congenital luxation of the hip was treated by manipulation, which he called "bloodless reduction," and he decried the traumatic method used by Lorenz and Lange in Europe. After reduction, he secured both limbs in the "frog" position in a plaster-of-paris cast whether only one hip was involved or not.

TENDONS

Murphy's interest in tendon surgery was mainly in corrective operations for congenital and acquired contractures. He employed both tenoplasty and tendon transplants along with neuroplasties and even arthrodesis in treating such lesions.

Tendon-lengthening procedures were described for talipes equinovarus, for the sequellae of cerebral palsy, and in a patient who had an obstetrical palsy from a long delivery with prolonged pressure on the sacral plexus that resulted in contractures at the knee and ankle. In another patient with contractures at the ankle and knee following a large hematoma in the leg, he lengthened the Achilles, gracilis, sartorius, semimembranosis, and semitendinosis tendons

In Volkmann's contractures he carefully dissected free the involved tendons, lengthened them appropriately by a double L incision, joined end-to-end the long limb of each L, and did an anterior capsulotomy at the elbow, even shortening the ulna and radius if necessary to let the tendons reach. He staggered the tendon suture lines and covered the areas with neighboring soft tissues to prevent agglutination. On occasion he even added arthroplasties where indicated. The more complex operations were sometimes staged (fig. 6.21).

He used tendon transplants to correct functional losses or deformities in poliomyelitis (fig. 6.22). If there was not enough tendon to use locally, Murphy would use the long flexors in the forearm as grafts. In a patient with substantial loss of the tibialis anticus muscle he used a tube of fascia lata to compensate for it (fig. 6.23). In a trauma patient who lost skin, fat, and tendons at the wrist, he covered the acute defect with a flap from the abdominal wall and in two later operations reattached the tendons.

In an instance of chronic tenovaginitis of the extensor of the thumb, he excised the tendon sheath and fashioned a new one out of pedicled flaps of fat. For tuberculous tenosynovitis, he made three injections of a modified Calot's solution at weekly intervals. This solution was prepared twenty-four hours ahead of time and consisted of the following: 1 percent formalin, 2 percent creosote, 2 percent guaiacol, and 95 percent glycerin or olive oil. To this was added by weight 10 percent of iodoform.

Murphy was truly a pioneer in orthopedic surgery. While the amount of orthopedic work he did was far less than the amount of general surgery, his innovations and contributions in this area were proportionately far greater. This was probably because the risks of bone and joint surgery were less life-threatening at the time than those that accompanied entering the abdomen or thorax.

REFERENCES

1. "Great moments in Illinois medicine," *Illinois Medicine* (May 11, 1990).

2. Petty, W., *Total Joint Replacement* (Philadelphia: Saunders, 1991), 6.

7

THORACIC SURGERY

Frank J. Milloy

While Murphy did relatively little thoracic surgery on patients, he did significant experimental work on animals in this field. This work was in part the basis for the surgical oration he was invited to give in 1898 at the annual meeting of the American Medical Association to be held in Denver, Colorado. In those days, at the annual AMA convention, a distinguished surgeon and an internist were each invited to give an oration summarizing the past year's progress in their respective fields.

In the introduction to his oration, Murphy alluded to Keen's address of the preceding year, which had summarized fifty years of progress in surgery. Rather than add one more year to that excellent recapitulation, Murphy chose to depart from the usual format and to present an overview of a single field of surgery—that of the lung. This was a subject he felt had not received as much attention as had surgery of the skeletal, nervous, or other systems.

The oration on surgery was given at the general session of the meeting rather than before a specialty group. Murphy's address was scheduled for the third day of the meeting. His was the only scientific presentation of the morning and was preceded by miscellaneous business. This was probably just as well as the address with lantern slides was exceedingly long and must have lasted well into the lunch hour.

According to accounts (2; 6), it was a distinct honor for Murphy at the age of forty-one to be selected by the doctors of the entire country to give the annual AMA oration. He undoubtedly believed that he would at last be accorded the much-desired respect of his fellow surgeons in Chicago as a result of this recognition. Little did he imagine the renewed criticism and personal attacks that would result because of a seemingly minor aspect of his oration, and the way it was publicized in the popular press.

ANNUAL SURGICAL ORATION

The address (JBM 54), which was a monograph on the subject of thoracic surgery, was a major scientific contribution. In his historic review, Murphy began in the fourth century B.C. with surgical drainage of a lung abscess, as described by Hippocrates. He then listed forty scientific references dating as far back as 1584, with authors such as Willis and Koch, up to the time of his contemporaries, who included Christian Fenger and E. Willis Andrews. The oration was divided into four subjects: anatomy, physiology, lung surgery, and experimental investigations.

Anatomy

The presentation of thoracic anatomy compared favorably with present-day teaching with a few exceptions. As an example of the latter, he stated that the tight garments of females deformed the thoracic cage into a balloon shape. Among the lantern slides Murphy used in illustrating thoracic anatomy were twelve chest roentgenograms. It is interesting to realize that a roentgenographic laboratory was in full operation in Chicago this soon after Roentgen's landmark discovery. The lantern slides that Murphy showed may well have been the first chest roentgenograms that many of the audience had ever seen. As late as 1908, a pulmonary lobectomy was performed in a Philadelphia hospital without the benefit of a roentgenogram of the chest because the hospital did not have the equipment (6).

Murphy noted that the lungs occupy only a fraction of the thoracic cavity because of the high dome of the diaphragm, which may rise as high as the level of the fourth interspace. He mentioned that the location of the internal mammary arteries make them susceptible to fatal hemorrhage. He described a procedure in which a thoracentesis needle was inserted at a low level into the chest. Serous fluid from the pleural space was withdrawn first. Then the needle was passed through the diaphragm and into the abdomen to yield pus from a subphrenic abscess. Thus, an important anatomic fact was illustrated, namely, the oblique configuration of the diaphragm, which at its posterior attachment often lies in a more vertical than transverse plane.

Physiology

There followed a comprehensive review of the physiological features of respiration in which he attributed the discovery of the true function of respiration to Mayow and cited a reference to the "Philisophical Transactions," London, 1666. Murphy quoted values for external spirometry that correspond to the values still recognized ninety years later. He pointed out that tidal volume during exercise reaches 366 cc of air but that vital capacity in forced respiration is almost ten times that volume. He also noted that patients with complete lung collapse due to massive pleural effusion still have respiratory exchange sufficient to sustain life. He therefore concluded that with sufficiently developed technic it would be possible to remove an entire lung. The first one-stage pneumonectomy would be performed thirty-five years later, by Evarts Graham in 1933 (3). Murphy recognized the importance of oxygen diffusion and gave the alveolar or diffusion surface of the lungs as 90 square meters.

Pneumothorax and Trauma

Murphy noted that the fear of creating pneumothorax was the greatest barrier to the development of surgery of the chest. In animal experiments he had found that the lung on the opened side of the chest gradually contracted to the hilum and that the mediastinal septum flapped to and fro "like a sail during a lull." If this situation was not remedied the animal died. He then quoted personal experiences with patients during operations or chest trauma in which the chest was opened. He found that grasping the collapsed lung with a forceps and pulling it into the opening in the chest wall immediately relieved the dyspnea; he thought this might be because the mediastinal septum was stabilized by such a maneuver. He also noted that suturing the lung to the margins of the chest-wall opening was effective.

Murphy stated that it was seldom necessary to treat spontaneous pneumothorax unless a valvular mechanism produced a positive pressure (tension pneumothorax), in which instance he advised making an incision in the ninth interspace beneath the tip of the scapula to relieve the pressure. He did not have the concept of closed chest drainage with water seal as we know it today. He also stated that "idiopathic pneumothorax" was due principally to tuberculosis and that 3 to 8 percent of tubercular patients would develop pneumothorax. This misconception was widely held for the next fifty or sixty years in some quarters, probably because spontaneous pneumothorax (which is due to ruptured pulmonary blebs, usually unrelated to tuberculosis) commonly occurs in the same young age group that is afflicted with pulmonary tuberculosis.

In discussing gunshot wounds to the chest, Murphy stated that he had gained great experience from patients seen in the emergency wards of Cook County Hospital. He noted that wounds involving the periphery of the lungs as a rule were not serious. If, however, there was evidence of bleeding from the internal mammary or intercostal arteries, or if evidence of late infection arose, these cases required surgical intervention.

Lung Abscess

Murphy discussed physical diagnosis of lung abscess at great length but did not mention roentgenographic findings. He enumerated the dangers of "exploratory puncture" for diagnosis of lung abscess and concluded that it would not become a common procedure. He stated that punctures and aspiration as treatment of lung abscess had fallen into disuse. To him it seemed preferable to make a large free opening in the chest wall by resection of portions of ribs, and then to open the lung cavity and allow free drainage.

Great effort was made to determine whether adhesions were present before open lung operations were attempted. Murphy thought that careful examination might reveal a pleural rub, which would mean a free pleural space. He described a method of introducing a trocar with a bag of sterile air attached. If there were no adhesions, air would flow into the chest cavity as the lung collapsed. In the presence of adhesions, however, there would be no air flow and the trocar would pass on into the lung substance.

Murphy stated that "irrigation of pulmonary cavities is rapidly going into disuse because it produces unpleasant symptoms." He cites the case of another surgeon in which the boric acid and thymol that were used for irrigation of a lung cavity resulted in death due to laryngobronchitis, and another instance in which a patient "almost drowned." In a twenty-year review of the literature from 1878 to 1897, Murphy collected 71 cases of lung abscess with 49 complete recoveries after operation, and 16 deaths. He then presented brief case histories of all 71 cases.

Bronchiectasis

Murphy gave a summary of the clinical and pathologic aspects of bronchiectasis. He felt that "universal" or widespread bronchiectasis was not a surgical disease, but that localized ampular bronchiectasis should be drained. After removal of two ribs (presumably the pleural space is obliterated by adhesions) "the sacular area of bronchiectasis is identified by means of palpation, or the exploratory needle. The lung parenchyma is then incised, the cavity entered, evacuated of pus, and packed open with iodoform gauze."

He performed this operation upon a forty-eight-year-old woman at

Cook County Hospital. After brief improvement, the patient died a month later. Postmortem examination revealed numerous "bronchial cavities" throughout the remaining lung tissue. Murphy thought his error had been in mistaking widespread disease for localized disease. These diagnoses were evidently made on the basis of physical findings that are minutely described in these case histories and seem over-interpreted by our standards today. He only mentioned roentgeno-graphic studies briefly. Bronchoscopy, and of course bronchography, were unknown to him. He summarized the case histories of forty-nine patients who had undergone operations for bronchiectatic cavities, found in a review of the literature, from 1873 to 1898.

Gangrene of the Lung

This entity was attributed to acute pneumonia in which the lung pa-renchyma instead of healing becomes necrotic. Murphy stated that when the prostration, intoxication, and "typhoid mutterings" con-tinue beyond the usual period for a pneumonia, gangrene must be suspected. He noted "there is probably no odor so offensive as that of the breath of a patient with gangrene of the lung." Murphy quoted a surgical dictum of the day: "Extensive gangrene cannot be cured by [conservative measures]; free incision should be made when gangrene is diagnosticated; operation is the only therapeutic efficient." He ad-vocated a large incision with free drainage. He stated that the compli-cations that arise in operations for gangrene are pneumothorax and hemorrhage. In the former case, the lung should be harpooned or grasped by a forceps and sutured to the wound edge. He presented a review of the world literature of ninety-six cases of patients who un-derwent operations for gangrene from 1879 to 1897, in addition to two more complete case histories of patients on whom he had oper-ated successfully.

Foreign Bodies

The foreign bodies enumerated as most common by Murphy are sur-prisingly similar to those seen today. He advocated taking advantage of gravity early in the problem before bronchoedema had fixed the foreign body in place. The patient was held by the feet, required to cough, and slapped on the chest with expiration. This was effective, he stated, in 60 percent of cases. Tracheostomy was used successfully in some cases. He felt that primary thoracotomy and bronchotomy were not justified because the percentage of cases in which the foreign body was found was small. He tells of a series of eleven cases mentioned by Tuffier in which there were four immediate deaths and in only one was the foreign body recovered.

Tuberculosis

There was great interest in pulmonary tuberculosis, one of the common causes of death in that era. Murphy emphasized the physical findings in all tuberculosis patients for evaluating the location and severity of their disease, but he also commonly employed chest roentgenograms even at this early date. He stated that "the x-ray is of inestimable value in studying pathologic processes of the lung, particularly in the localization of cavities. The degree of compression of the lung can be photographed and the rapidity of the absorption of gas estimated by comparison of pictures" (JBM 54). We see an early appreciation of the value of serial roentgenograms in following the course of the disease.

As explained in Chapter 10, Murphy favored collapse therapy for cavitary tuberculosis but he also used open drainage and packing. He described a patient in whom he removed the anterior three inches of the second and third ribs through a U-shaped skin incision and then separated the pleura from the chest wall for a distance of one inch around the field of operation. He then made an exploratory puncture to locate the cavity and opened into the cavity at about a depth of one inch. Hemorrhage was not profuse and after digital exploration of the cavity he packed it open with iodoform gauze. The skin flap was sutured around the drain. The patient did well (JBM 54, p. 341).

Murphy presented a review of the literature in which there were 47 operations performed for tuberculosis between 1878 and 1898. Incision and drainage were performed in 34, thoracoplasty in 5, opening of a superficial abscess in 4, puncture drainage in 2, and "pneumectomy" in 2. There were 28 recoveries and 19 deaths.

Murphy categorized the removal of any lung tissue under the heading of "pneumectomy." He stated that the removal of a complete lobe of the lung or part of a lobe for tuberculous disease had been one of the triumphs of surgical technic, but so far the clinical results had been unsatisfactory. "From [previous experimental studies] we were led to believe that pneumectomy as a curative method for tuberculous lesions of the lung would become an acceptable surgical procedure; however, our hopes have not been realized. While the operation of removal of a complete lobe of a lung has been successfully performed the number of deaths following pneumectomy have been so large that the operation has been practically abandoned."

He cites three surgeons from the literature—Tuffier in 1891, Lowson in 1893, and Doyen in 1895—as having performed "pneumectomies" for tuberculosis successfully. Tuffier removed a "piece of lung 2 cm in all directions" through an incision in the second interspace in a twenty-year-old male. The wound was closed without drainage; the patient was up on the ninth day and was healthy four years after the operation.

Murphy noted a problem still vexing surgeons today, that "the pathologic conditions which render these operations necessary are such that at a time most favorable for the performance of the operations the patient will not submit. But when they desire the operation because of the symptoms, the pathologic changes are so far advanced that they are not in condition to withstand its severity." He then enumerated the structures of the chest which may be damaged in freeing a lobe and stated that the ligature must be placed at the base of the lobe including only the artery, veins, and bronchi, and that the chest incision must be sufficiently large to permit the extraction of a mass the size of a lobe. He appears to have planned to use a single mass ligature for lobectomy through an anterior incision.

Murphy stated that "the removal of a complete lung for tuberculosis has not to my knowledge been attempted. In advanced tuberculosis the pathologic changes produce insurmountable barriers against the operation of pneumectomy and while occasional success in partial resections may be achieved it can never become a practical method for the treatment of tuberculosis." This inaccurate prediction is reminiscent of the admonition attributed to Billroth that the human heart would never be amenable to surgical operations.

Neoplasm

Murphy stated that primary malignant neoplasms of the lung were rare, but that secondary (metastatic) involvement by carcinoma and sarcoma were not uncommon. "In many cases it is difficult to say whether malignant disease is primary or secondary in the lung; the surgeon is rarely called upon to operate on these cases as they are not diagnosed." The class of malignant disorders of the lung which came to the surgeon for operation was that in which a tumor of the chest wall extended to involve the lung.

He noted that "the first pneumectomy was made by Pean in 1861." He was resecting a chest-wall tumor involving three ribs when the lung was found adherent and involved in the tumor. The Paquelin cautery was used to remove the diseased portion of lung.

In a review of the literature from 1884 to 1896, Murphy found six patients who had undergone operations for chest-wall sarcomata with lung invasion, five involving ribs and one of the sternum. The lesions with portions of lung were all resected. Three patients survived and three died within hours of the operation, two of pneumothorax and one of "purulent pleurisy."

Besides the diseases mentioned above, there were short discussions of pulmonary actinomycosis and hydatid disease. He also discussed hernia of the lung and described a case published in 1492 by Rolandus of Bologna in which the herniated portion of the lung was amputated. He considered this the first recorded case of partial lung resection. He did not consider the amputation of a herniating part of the lung to be a true "pneumectomy," however, because it did not involve the dangers and difficulties of technic associated with intrathoracic operations.

Experimental Surgery

Murphy described several experimental lobectomies and a pneumonectomy he had performed in dogs. These resections were accomplished using a mass ligature technic at the hilus. There was one long-term survivor after lobectomy in whom extensive postmortem microscopic examination demonstrated the healing process of the vessels and bronchus.

In this series of ten animal experiments, he made several notable observations that still pertain to lung surgery today. He found the fifth rib level ideal for entry into the thorax because it permitted easy access to the hilus of the lung. He also attempted to cover the bronchial stump with a flap of pleura, following resection. Finally, he aspirated air from the operated side after the pneumonectomy, to pull the mediastinum over and permit full use of the remaining lung.

In his last experiment, a large dog was described as difficult to anesthetize and cardiopulmonary arrest occurred when the chest was opened. A tracheostomy was performed and a rubber tube inserted into the trachea. The air passages were occluded around the tube and the lung could easily be made to expand. This, according to Murphy, illustrated "Tuffier's method of artificial respiration."

Summary

Murphy's monograph was an exhaustive review of the basic anatomy and physiology of the thorax and breathing apparatus that was largely identical to what we understand today. There followed an extensive review of the history and of the practice of lung surgery up to

1898. With each specific disease there was a list of brief case histories of patients undergoing operations collected from the recent world literature. There were also included a few case histories of patients on whom Murphy himself had operated.

The operations described from the literature were almost all "pneumotomies" for the incision and drainage of lung abscesses, tuberculous cavities, and bronchiectatic cavities. He reserved the term "pneumectomy" for the actual removal of lung tissue. Although he had not performed a pneumectomy himself, he described cases done by others. In these cases a relatively small amount of lung (what would now be termed a "wedge") had been removed.

The references throughout Murphy's paper were listed in the body of the text or at the bottom of the page. If a standard bibliography had been appended at the end of the paper, it would have consisted of hundreds of items.

The oration with illustrations required fifty-three pages of double-column small print for publication in the *Journal of the American Medical Association,* where it appeared in four consecutive installments from July 23 to August 13, 1898. The first installment appeared only a month after the oration was delivered.

The oration was well written, with only minor errors immediately apparent. Murphy gave two different dates for Rolandus's pioneering lung amputation and he described Doyen's pneumectomy as a success in one place and stated in another that the patient died the night of the operation.

Considering the extreme length of the text and the fact that Murphy was said to be a poor speaker with a high-pitched voice and a too-rapid delivery, it must have been difficult to follow. According to records (2; 4), however, the oration was received enthusiastically by the assembled physicians and surgeons and he was extended a vote of thanks for his able and instructive presentation.

Murphy's understanding of the essential anatomy and physiology was remarkable, as was his very extensive review of the literature. His use of the limited surgical methods of his day reveal a basic conservatism but also a willingness to undertake the management of difficult surgical problems. The animal experiments, though limited in number, were exactly in line toward the development of the technic of lung resection which would be achieved in the ensuing forty years. The delivery of this landmark summary of lung surgery at the turn of the century brought the American profession up to date on this subject both in historical perspective and current clinical and experimental applications.

HISTORICAL PERSPECTIVE

The oration helps to answer three pertinent questions: How did the lung disease of Murphy's day compare to that which we encounter at present? What was the state of the surgical art at that time? To what degree had Murphy himself contributed to lung surgery at the turn of the century?

Nature of Pulmonary Diseases—Then and Now

Aside from trauma, the nature of human pathology differed greatly at the turn of the century from what we commonly see today. As for trauma, Murphy had stated in his address that there were many patients with stab wounds and gunshot wounds of the chest in the emergency wards of Cook County Hospital with a great variety of pathological manifestations. That is still true today.

On the other hand, largely due to the introduction of antibiotic drugs, profound changes have taken place in the nature of pulmonary pathology in America since Murphy's time. Whereas improved sanitation in the 1800s had begun to eliminate the plagues of cholera and typhoid (1), it was not until the 1930s and 1940s that the introduction of the broad-spectrum antibiotics made it possible to cure more successfully the common pneumonias. One result has been that bronchiectasis, which Murphy found highly prevalent, and which is the result of repeated lung infections, has almost been eliminated as an indication for surgical management. This is also true of lung abscess, a more acute complication of pneumonia. The infections are now treated at an early stage with antibiotics. Bronchiectasis and lung abscess do not have an opportunity to develop or, if they do develop, are more easily controlled with the antibiotics.

A second advance was the antituberculous drugs introduced in the 1950s. Tuberculosis, which in Murphy's time was one of the commonest causes of death, was so contagious and so financially devastating that, throughout the country, a network of special sanitaria had been built by local governments for the free care of thousands of chronically ill tuberculous patients. Whereas at one time Chicago's municipal tuberculosis sanitarium had as many as fifteen hundred beds, at present there is no longer a sanitarium in the Chicago area, and as a result of modern infection control, tuberculosis is almost a rare disease among American-born patients.

Because of the infectious diseases, life expectancy was only forty-seven years for a child born in 1900 and people did not commonly live into the cancer age as they do today. There are undoubtedly other factors involved, but for whatever reason, as Murphy stated, primary lung cancer was indeed a rare disease. The few malignancies he does describe are chest-wall sarcomata with lung invasion, a tumor of younger patients.

Since Murphy's time, then, as a result of antibiotics, the chronic lung infections have been practically eliminated. At least twenty years have been added to life expectancy and Americans have been brought into the age group where lung cancer, far from being a rare disease, is now one of the commonest causes of death. As a corollary, the presence or even the suspicion of primary lung cancer is now a far more common indication for operation than a lung infection.

Lung Surgery at the Turn of the Century

Surgical specialization as we know it today did not exist in the 1800s. The American Association of Thoracic Surgery was not founded until 1916 and the *Journal of Thoracic Surgery* was first published in 1931. Some surgeons of the 1800s were more interested than others in lung operations, among whom Tuffier of France was a capable and innovative pioneer. Stephen Paget's *The Surgery of the Chest* (7), a 470-page text published in 1896 in London, was, according to the author, the first book in English on the subject. Paget stated that Mr. Godlee was "the pioneer of English surgeons in [this] great field of practice, which during the last five and twenty years, thanks to Lister, has advanced with wonderful rapidity."

Paget's book was published in New York only a few months before Murphy's oration. However, Murphy had read it and quoted it as his source for Rolandus's case of lung hernia. Perhaps it was in part the inspiration for Murphy's choice of lung surgery as the topic of his oration. At any rate, the fact of its publication indicated the growing interest in this field of surgery. As to the state of the art of thoracic surgery in Murphy's day, it was on the threshold of remarkable progress.

Empyema Drainage. Intrathoracic collections of pus had been drained since the time of Hippocrates, either by simple incision or the use of cannulas. By the 1800s it was recognized that the entrance of air into the chest in the course of empyema drainage was often undesirable. With the invention of rubber tubing, closed chest drainage, as we know it today, became practicable.

In his exhaustive history of thoracic surgery before the twentieth century, Hochberg (4) credits Thomas Davis in 1835 as introducing a "gum-elastic catheter . . . into the chest" through which fluid was evacuated intermittently. Potain in 1869 described a syphon apparatus to prevent air from entering the chest in the course of thoracocentesis. Finally, Playfair of England in 1872 described an apparatus in which "the drainage tube lies within the cavity of the pleura [and is attached to] an india rubber tube [that] passes through a perforated cork into a bottle half filled with water." This was very similar to the simple closed-chest drainage water-seal bottle in use today.

Operations on the Lung. It would seem from Murphy's paper that not many lung operations had been performed. In his extensive review of the recent world literature he had found 71 operations for lung abscess, 49 for bronchiectatic cavity, and 95 for what he termed gangrene. These were almost all anecdotal experiences, gathered from individual case reports. There were apparently no large series. These operations were almost all pneumonotomies, simple procedures to drain pus. The surgeon upon entering the pleura hoped that adhesions would be present, whereupon he dissected or cauterized through lung tissue until he reached the abscess (if he could find it), which he then evacuated of pus and packed open. If the surgeon made the incision and no adhesions were present, the lung then collapsed, more or less completely, and the mediastinum began to swing with each respiration, which of course could be fatal. As noted above, Murphy advised in this situation that the lung be grasped with an instrument and pulled into the wound, thus preventing the entrance of air and stabilizing the mediastinum. Obviously under these circumstances, a careful dissection at the root of the lung to isolate the vessels and perform a modern type of lung resection would have been impossible.

The concept of positive pressure anesthesia, which makes present-day lung surgery easy, was only just arriving. Even when the patient made it through the operation, the chest was closed tightly and sometimes it was simply reported that the individual died hours later of pneumothorax.

Murphy's Contribution

As to Murphy's own contributions to lung surgery, they too can best be described as anecdotal. In his oration he did not present a formal list of his patients but interposed in his discussion brief case histories of people he had treated. There were two gunshot wounds, an open drainage of a tuberculous bronchiectatic cavity, drainage of two cases of gangrene of the lung, thoracoplasty for a tuberculous cavity, drainage of a tuberculous cavity, and open drainage for hydatid disease.

There were also five cases of artificial pneumothorax for tuberculosis, which will be discussed later.

Murphy's major efforts in thoracic surgery occurred in his laboratory. In one of his *Surgical Clinic* discussions (*SC* 234) he advises that after experimental surgery on arteries and veins one should turn to the lung,

> open the chest wall and transplant the lung through the ribs by spreading and resecting them. Read the technical feats which have been accomplished and do them; then do the things which have not yet been done. Remember, the surgery of the lung has been one of the slowest fields to be cultivated, chiefly on account of the bugbear of pneumothorax. This bugbear is almost a myth, and yet you all hear about it, and every student goes out of college having a horror of it. Do you know that the first removal of a lung on record was performed by a bull in Bologna nearly five hundred years ago? If a bull could extract a lung and the patient's life be saved, why should not a surgeon do it? That case is an actual historic fact.

He then recounts the details of Rolandus's case.

Murphy performed a pneumonectomy on a dog by passing a massive ligature around the entire hilus of the lung, which included pulmonary artery, veins, and bronchus. This is the same technic employed by Evarts Graham, when in 1933 he performed the first successful one-stage pneumonectomy. Graham stated that the hilus was doubly ligated en masse with transfixing ligatures of chromic catgut after separate ligation of the pulmonary artery (3).

Interestingly, in the last animal experiment Murphy described he performed a tracheostomy and forced air into the dog's lungs. As mentioned earlier, he referred to this as the method of Tuffier. Hochberg tells that Tuffier and Hallion in 1896 suggested endotrachial intubation and the delivery of positive pressure to the lung. Murphy observed how little pressure was required for the lung to expand and protrude out of the chest cavity.

It would seem that if Murphy had done a few more animal experiments he might have combined the method of positive pressure anesthesia of Tuffier with the apparatus of closed chest drainage devised by Playfield and then been on the way to lung surgery as we know it today. It is unfortunate that he had not the laboratory facilities of a present-day surgical department at that point in his career.

The one concept in the entire oration that Murphy considered an original contribution was in the management of pulmonary tuberculosis. He recalled the principle of putting injured or diseased parts of the body at rest to promote healing, and also the desirability to cause tubercular cavities to collapse so that the walls might heal together. He stated that this might be accomplished by the injection of nitrogen gas into the pleural space, thus creating a limited pneumothorax. He described how he had performed this procedure in eight patients, in three of whom it was unsuccessful because of adhesions that prevented lung collapse.

This one, rather minor aspect of the oration was to be sensationalized and was to bring his name to prominence in ways he would regret. The day after Murphy delivered the oration, Friday, June 10, the story was reported on the front page of the *Chicago Tribune,* under the following headlines:

SAYS HE CURES CONSUMPTION
Dr. J. B. Murphy of Chicago Addressed
The American Medical Association in Denver

HOW TO TREAT THE LUNG
Collapses the Organ by Nitrogen Gas Injected
Through a Needle in the Pleural Space
QUICK SUCCESS IN FIVE CASES

NATURE USES PLEURITIS EFFUSION TO HEAL
THE DISEASED MEMBER WHILE IT RESTS FROM
ITS WORK

COUNTY HOSPITAL TRIALS COMING

The account was continued on page seven in two columns, with a two-column picture of Murphy (2). Of course this enraged his colleagues in Chicago. The fact that the story had appeared so promptly after the oration, and in such sensational form, made many suspicious that he had sought the publicity and may have himself, or through others, given the story to the newspaper.

But this was only the beginning. Murphy said later, "When I returned to Chicago I found my room packed three feet deep with mail from persons who asked about the treatment. The first time in my life that I was ever frightened was when I saw that massive mail" (2). One can imagine the reaction this publicity had caused in those unfortunate individuals who were dying of tuberculosis. A second criticism came later along more professional lines. Forlanini, an Italian surgeon, had published the technic of artificial pneumothorax in an Italian journal several years previously. Murphy's failure to acknowledge Forlanini's work would be used against him for years.

MURPHY AND LUNG SURGERY AFTER THE SURGICAL ORATION

What was Murphy's interest in lung surgery after 1898? This was the period of the most important advance in lung surgery made up to that time—the introduction of positive pressure endotracheal anesthesia. As mentioned, Murphy had used this technic in the laboratory.

In William Mushin's *Thoracic Anesthesia* (8), Rendell-Baker described the Fell-O'Dwyer apparatus as a laryngeal intubating cannula attached to a foot-operated bellows for positive pressure respiration, which had been developed for the management of diphtheria. He quotes Tuffier and Hallion in 1896 and Matas in 1899 as recognizing its value for the performance of lung resections. Rendell-Baker attributed to Parham, an associate of Matas, the first use of this device in a thoracotomy. Parham (1899) believed the apparatus would revolutionize the field of thoracic surgery, making possible operations in the chest that would otherwise be clearly too hazardous.

Had Murphy been solely interested in lung surgery, this should have been a time of increased activity. With the advantage of endotracheal anesthesia and a quiet operative field he might have performed on a human the lobectomy or even pneumonectomy he had performed in the animal laboratory.

It was not Murphy alone, however, who was reluctant to undertake lung operations. Although Tuffier and Hallion agreed with Matas and Parham in the 1890s that positive pressure endotracheal anesthesia would solve the main problem of open-chest operations, there was no great increase in the number of these procedures.

Some attribute the failure of endotracheal anesthesia to gain popularity to the introduction by Sauerbruch in 1904 of his negative pressure chamber. In this apparatus the surgeon was in an air-tight compartment with the patient's torso while the patient's head protruded outside, an air-tight collar around the patient's neck preserving the seal. By raising and lowering the pressure inside the chamber rhythmically, the patient's lungs could be expanded and compressed and his blood oxygenated, with the chest opened. This permitted operations without the problem of lung collapse. Although the Sauerbruch chamber became popular in Europe, Willy Meyer of New York was evidently the only American surgeon to build one (6).

According to Mead (6), Gluck had performed lobectomies in 1899 and 1900, which were the first successfully carried out in humans. Meyer, however, in a paper read at the American Surgical Association in April of 1914, reported that his review of the world literature revealed that up to that time only sixteen lobectomies had been performed for bronchiectasis, with a 50 percent mortality.

In addition to the problems of anesthesia that required either the complicated Sauerbruch chamber or an anesthetist who could intubate the trachea and operate one of the complicated positive pressure machines of the day, there was still the problem of postoperative pneumothorax. Sauerbruch (6) reported doing three lobectomies in 1920 after which he closed the chest tightly without drainage; all three patients died of tension pneumothorax.

Considering the fact that Playfair and others had developed water-seal drainage as early as 1872, Mead states that "it is difficult to understand why our present system of under-water seal for closed drainage was not used in the early days." The first reference he could find to its routine usage was in 1922.

THE *SURGICAL CLINICS* RECORDS

The *Surgical Clinics* volumes contain over seven hundred operations done largely by Murphy, but only a handful relate to thoracic surgery and these we will briefly review in chronological order:

Sarcoma of the thymus gland (*SC* 179): A sixty-nine-year-old female presented with a slowly enlarging mass over the sternum of twenty years duration. Murphy aspirated the mass and obtained bright red blood. He concluded that this represented an aneurysmal sarcoma of the sternum rather than a thymoma and advocated radiation treatment in preference to operation.

Tuberculosis of the lung; production of artificial penumothorax by injection of nitrogen according to Dr. Murphy's method (*SC* 192): A thirty-two-year-old female with a one-year history of tuberculosis was presented. She had undergone two intrapleural injections of nitrogen, one ten days previously. No treatment was given, but Murphy used the opportunity for a lengthy discussion of pulmonary tuberculosis. He stated that since 1898 his associates had used artificial pneumothorax in 460 patients. He himself had not done the procedure since the original eight cases he described in the surgical oration in 1898 because he felt it was more appropriate for internists to make the injections rather than surgeons.

Empyema (*SC* 221): A child was presented with postpneumonitic empyema. Murphy drew attention to finger clubbing as a sign of pleural disease. He then discussed at length the possible etiologies of empyema. He suggested a careful thoracentesis with a small needle and warned that perforation of the diaphragm may cause peritonitis. For treatment, free drainage is indicated in every type of empyema except tuberculous. The child was anesthetized, drainage performed, and a rubber drain sutured in place.

Intrathoracic sarcoma starting from the vertebral column (*SC* 279): A forty-seven-year-old male with a five-month history of back pain and X-ray findings of a right paravertebral chest mass was discussed. Murphy and his associate Dr. Charles Mix concluded that the lesion was a sarcoma arising from the spine and no operation was performed.

Carbuncle of the arm—septicemia—metastatic pleurisy—death (*SC* 326): A twenty-seven-year-old male with a two-week history of a carbuncle on the anterior angle of his shoulder extending into the axilla was toxic and dyspneic on admission. Murphy performed a wide-open drainage procedure on the carbuncle with incision down to fascia. The patient became more toxic and died forty-eight hours later. There was no mention of treatment of the empyema presumed present.

Tuberculosis of sternum and rib—excision and sinus curettage (*SC* 381): A forty-one-year-old woman presented with a draining sinus over the sternum. Six years previously she was operated upon for removal of cervical tuberculous lymphadenitis. A sinogram was shown. Murphy excised the sinus, the involved portion of the sternum, and the entire involved cartilage.

Bronchiectatic cavity—compression of lung (*SC* 383): A twenty-five-year-old male was presented with a ten-year history of cough and hemoptysis. Murphy incised to the parietal pleura in the seventh interspace where he noted that the lung was moving in a free pleural space and that there were therefore no adhesions. He then packed the interspace with nosophen gauze. Two days later, on September 28, 1914, he reopened the incision and removed a portion of rib, but he could still see movement of the lung, indicating that it would not be wise to open a lung cavity without adhesions present because the entire pleural space would then be contaminated. He did open the pleura, however, because he removed a pint of fluid and noted that the lung was fully collapsible. He then stated there was now "too much air in the pleural space" but that he would aspirate it.

Empyema of pleural cavity resection of ribs (Estlander) (*SC* 407): A thirty-eight-year-old male patient, who had a three-year history of draining chest sinus that followed rib resection for tuberculous empyema drainage, was presented. Murphy discussed empyema in adults and then performed a six-rib thoracoplasty. Six months post-operatively the wound had stopped draining and the patient had gained forty pounds.

Infective costal perichondritis—resection of costal cartilages (*SC* 503): A thirty-three-year-old male was seen by Murphy in February 1916. Two years before, while the man was sitting in a dental chair, the drill had dropped to his chest and wounded the patient over the left fifth rib, three inches from the sternum. Over the ensuing months the patient had undergone several drainage procedures of his left anterior chest. Murphy thought that the etiology of the infection was from mouth organisms rather than tuberculosis or typhoid, the usual causes of such lesions. Through an extensive "vest-flap" incision, the left seventh and eighth cartilages were completely removed, the sinuses were laid open, and all granulation tissue was curetted.

Sarcoma of sternum—resection (*SC* 544): A sixty-year-old female was admitted with a slightly tender, hard swelling over the upper sternum, one-half inch in diameter. Through a "vest-flap" incision a tumor of the manubrium of the sternum was excised locally. On pathologic examination this proved to be a giant-cell sarcoma.

Sinus of abdomen from gangrene of lung—celiotomy with drainage (*SC* 605): A twenty-five-year-old male patient developed a chronic draining sinus of the right lower quadrant following an appendectomy. A sinogram was performed (by means of injecting bismuth), and Murphy interpreted it as showing a subphrenic abscess. Through a subcostal incision Murphy traced the sinus tract through the diaphragm into the chest. He concluded that the patient had originally had gangrene of the lung, which had presented as appendicitis and then drained through the abdomen. Although he did not give a pathologic diagnosis on removed tissue, Murphy notes that the patient made an uneventful recovery.

These eleven patients seen by Murphy from 1912 until his death in 1916 are evidently the only thoracic surgical cases that came under his care during that period. They do not include his most famous patient, former president Theodore Roosevelt, who was shot in the chest on October 12, 1912, in Milwaukee and brought to Chicago for care by Murphy, as discussed in Chapter 1. Roosevelt's wound was only superficial, however, and did not require operative intervention. In only one case, the attempted drainage of a "bronchiectatic cavity" (*SC* 383), did Murphy actually enter the free pleural space.

The introduction of the cuffed endotracheal tube in America is generally attributed to Janeway in 1913 (8), advancing the contributions of Tuffier and Fell, previously mentioned. But in September 1914 Murphy was obviously doing a thoracotomy in the presence of a free pleural space without an endotracheal tube or even positive pressure anesthesia (*SC* 383).

He performed the operation in the accepted two-stage manner as then advocated. According to the theory, in the first stage an incision was made down to the parietal pleura. If the lung could be seen to move with respiration (through the transparent parietal pleura) the incision was carried no farther and irritating material (iodoform gauze) was packed into the wound in the hope that adhesions would have formed between the two pleural layers when the incision was reopened several days later. Then, at the time of reoperation, incision in the lung could be performed without the occurrence of a pneumothorax.

In this case, however, the first stage had not produced the desired adhesions and at the second operation there was still a free pleural space. Nevertheless, Murphy proceeded to open the chest in order to produce a pneumothorax so that the lung and therefore the bronchiectatic cavity would collapse and be more amenable to healing. This was good theory, except that Murphy was then faced with a total pneumothorax and collapsed lung. He must have been working through a small incision because he was evidently able to achieve an air-tight seal around an aspirator and reexpand the lung. How he kept the lung expanded during the closure is not explained. There is no record that he ever used water-seal drainage.

One can only marvel at Murphy—with only drop ether anesthesia available—opening the pleural space, producing a total pneumothorax, and then calmly remarking to the audience that he had asked for the aspirator to be ready for just such an emergency—and this when he was suffering from angina pectoris.

Finally, it should be mentioned that Murphy was interested in an early pulmotor. He describes its use postoperatively in a young patient with an inoperable cerebellar tumor who had stopped breathing and whom he kept alive for thirty-four hours by means of the machine. However, he felt, "the pulmotor is too expensive a machine for common use, but we are working out a plan to run it for 3 per cent. of what it costs to run it now. By referring to the article on the Surgery of the Lung that I wrote in 1898, you will find that I showed that more than 3 per cent. of oxygen in the air is an absolute waste; . . . therefore you can use 3 per cent. of additional oxygen and 97 per cent. of compressed air and get apparently the same results" (*SC* 174).

Perhaps the most interesting aspect of these reports is the informal nature of the discussion. Murphy's comments were transcribed verbatim as he lectured and operated, and as the amount of repetition would seem to indicate, they were printed with very little editing. As a result, the reader gains an intimate impression of Murphy and his personality, and of the nature of the practice of surgery in that era.

PAPERS ON TUBERCULOSIS IN 1914

After his "Oration on Surgery of the Lung" in 1898, Murphy did not write about tuberculosis again until 1914 when two papers were published. One was coauthored by Kreuscher (JBM 132) and appeared in the *Interstate Medical Journal*. The other was a transcript of a talk given at the Chicago Medical Society (JBM 131). This talk took place on the evening of January 7, 1914, at a symposium on tuberculosis, part of a regular meeting of the Chicago Medical Society. Murphy was the third speaker, following Dr. Weiner and Dr. Gray. The talk was very informal and from the casual expressions used seems to have been totally ad lib rather than read from a prepared text.

In the talk he says that when he first advocated the injection of nitrogen into the chest in 1898 he did not know of previous investigators' works. Since then he had learned that this treatment was first advocated by Carson of Liverpool in 1822, who had created artificial pneumothoraces in rabbits, from which they recovered. Therefore, Carson felt that one lung could be collapsed with impunity and concluded that pulmonary tuberculosis could be treated by this mechanical means. Murphy noted that in the next forty-five years Parolo, Ramodge, Conslatt, Wunderlich, and Ehler all referred to Carson's theory but none had attempted the operation. Forlanini of Padua was next to write on the subject, in 1882, but Murphy understood that he had not actually performed the procedure. However, Hochberg (4) says that Carson and Forlanini had each submitted two patients to artificial pneumothorax but "it took the fame of Murphy . . . to awaken the medical world to the value of artificial pneumothorax in the management of pulmonary tuberculosis." Forlanini had presented his paper at the 1894 Surgical Congress in Rome, which Murphy attended as the official United States representative, but it should be noted that over three thousand papers were read at that congress and Murphy may well not have heard Forlanini's presentation (2).

Murphy stated that by this time, 1914, there had been 386 articles on artificial pneumothorax published in the literature. And he noted, "So far as we are able to find today, we were the first to use nitrogen in the practical compression of the lung. But priority means nothing.

The treatment which was suggested and published by me in my surgical oration in 1898 in Denver was not accepted by the American profession, and it is just a little pleasurable tonight to feel that that method [previously criticized] is now the dominant method of treatment of tuberculosis all over the world." Thus we obtain an insight into Murphy's personal feelings about this matter in which he evidently felt he had been wronged over the years by unfair criticism.

As to his own practice, he had 460 patients who had undergone some two thousand nitrogen injections by his associates. He stated that he had one complication, an air embolism that had produced hemiplegia. It is interesting that he recognized an embolism for what it was and was not confused by "pleural shock" or "vago-vagal reflexes" and the other nebulous terms which were popular in that day.

Then he compared his method of lung collapse to that of Friedrich's "colossal" operation of removing all of the ribs to allow the side to sink in and of Cobb who removed segments of ribs one through eight and of parts of the corresponding costal cartilages to permit a falling in the chest wall. He questioned that if these able men felt that it was justified to resort to these "terrific" operations to occlude cavities, why not use the simple insertion of a needle, which was practically free from danger.

These "terrific" operations Murphy referred to were of course the precursors of the three-stage seven-rib thoracoplasty that John Alexander would perfect in the 1930s and which along with artificial pneumothorax, each in its own place, would constitute the chief surgical therapy for pulmonary tuberculosis until the specific antituberculous drugs were introduced in the 1950s. These drugs, streptomycin, isoniazid, and para-aminosalicylic acid, which Murphy would have indeed considered miraculous, permitted the control of the disease and, along with improvements in anesthesia, allowed performance of the operations he thought would never be possible—lobectomy and pneumonectomy—to become routine in the management of pulmonary tuberculosis. Thus a concept he had expressed in his original oration—"the ideal treatment of tuberculosis is irradication; extirpation of the tubercular focus"—eventually came to be realized. It is unfortunate that he could not have witnessed it.

Murphy told of the doctors of Chicago first doing acid-fast stains in 1883, the year following Koch's discovery of the organism, and finding the bacilli much more frequently than they had suspected, so that patients who had initially been considered as merely bronchiatatic were then found to have tuberculosis. Before that the great clinicians would locate a lung cavity by ausculation and percussion and then announce that the patient had tuberculosis because the cavity was present.

We should recall that near the end of his fascinating if somewhat rambling paper, Murphy said, "Now for the local management of tuberculosis of the lung on which I was supposed to speak this evening." One wonders if he had completely ignored his prepared text and then later published it in the *Interstate Medical Journal.* The latter paper certainly corresponds to the title more closely than did the informal talk that he gave at the Chicago Medical Society that night.

The two papers that appeared sixteen years after his controversial 1898 oration on lung surgery, with little or nothing on pulmonary tuberculosis published in between, seemed almost an afterthought, as though he were mentally tying up a few loose ends. He would be dead of myocardial ischemia in less than three years and was already experiencing angina. Perhaps he had an inkling of what was to come and wanted to set the record straight while he was still able.

There has been speculation (6) as to why Murphy lost interest in pulmonary surgery after the famous oration. Several observations seem appropriate. Murphy had done only a few lung operations, and the oration seems to have been an exercise in self-education for Murphy himself, as much as anything. He did not show the great interest in lung surgery exhibited by others, Tuffier or Sauerbruch, for instance. Furthermore, as mentioned above, the failure of surgeons to adopt positive pressure anesthesia and closed-chest drainage for over twenty years after they were first described made lung surgery a formidable undertaking with a 50 percent mortality up until the 1920s.

Editors' note: Much of the preceding chapter is a modification of Dr. Milloy's article "The contributions of John B. Murphy to thoracic surgery," *Surg. Gynecol. Obstet.* 171 (1990): 421–32. It appears here by permission of *Surgery, Gynecology and Obstetrics.*

REFERENCES

1. Bonner, T., *Medicine in Chicago 1850–1950* (Madison, Wis.: American History Research Center, 1957).

2. Davis, L., *J. B. Murphy: Stormy Petrel of Surgery* (New York: Putnam, 1938).

3. Graham, E., and J. J. Singer, "Successful removal of an entire lung for carcinoma of the bronchus," *JAMA* 101 (1933): 1371–74.

4. Hochberg, L., *Thoracic Surgery before the 20th Century* (New York: Vantage, 1960).

5. Martin, F. H., *Fifty Years of Medicine and Surgery; an Autobiographi-*

cal Sketch (Chicago: Surgical Publishing Company of Chicago, 1934).

6. Mead, R. H., *A History of Thoracic Surgery* (Springfield, Ill.: Thomas, 1961).

7. Paget, S., *The Surgery of the Chest* (London: Simpkin, Marshall, Hamilton, Kent, 1896

8. Rendell-Baker, L., "History of the thoracic anesthesia," in *Thoracic Anesthesia*, ed. W. Mushin (Philadelphia: Davis, 1963).

9. Rutkow, I. M., "A history of the *Surgical Clinics of North America*," *Surg. Clin. North Am.* 67 (1987): 1217.

8

UROLOGY

James J. Burden, Eugene T. McEnery, and
Robert L. Schmitz

Although urologic surgery was in its infancy in the late nineteenth century, Murphy added it to his practice. Eleven of his journal articles deal with urological topics, and the *Surgical Clinics* describe forty-six separate urological operations. Occasionally the reports include a statistical review of his immediate results but long-term results are seldom mentioned.

KIDNEY AND URETER

The first nephrectomy was performed by Wolcott of Milwaukee in 1861 (4). By 1885, Sam Gross could review 233 nephrectomies from the literature, finding a mortality rate of 45 percent (3).

Murphy did his first operation on the kidney in 1888. It was a two-stage operation for a bad pyelonephritic kidney. The kidney was first drained posteriorly. At the second stage, performed transabdominally, there was still much induration and he had great difficulty freeing the kidney from the aorta and vena cava. Eventually he succeeded but he said "it was the most difficult operation I had ever performed" (JBM 27).

For the usual nephrectomy he accepted the posterior approach because it carried a lower mortality. However, in large renal masses he used an anterior route, going either extraperitoneally or transabdominally. The February 1895 records of a Cook County Hospital Alumni Association meeting include a discussion by Murphy of kidney sarcomas (very likely the lesion Wilms described in 1899) in which he recommended this route, saying, "I believe the method of attacking these tumors from behind will before long be surgery of the past" (5).

If the pedicle was difficult to expose, clamps were used instead of ligatures. These were left on for four or five days. The clamps had detachable handles (fig. 8.1) and the shafts were tied tightly with gauze to prevent premature unlocking (*SC* 228, p. 326). They were positioned with the tips pointing forward so that a simple backward movement could remove them without pulling on the pedicle.

During a nephrectomy for a suppurating cystic kidney he tore into the vena cava. Murphy recalled, "In looking at it I simply put on three hemostats, went on with my enucleation upward from that, and did an overstitch of the vena cava." The patient survived (*SC* 47).

In pursuing renal calculi, he was not afraid to open the renal pelvis and inspect the inside of the kidney. This was considered inadvisable by other surgeons, including Christian Fenger (*SC* 68). If the stone was lower in the ureter, he did ureterotomy, then closed the ureter and placed a small drain that was sewn to the skin and removed after ten days (*SC* 127; 412; 549).

Murphy was among the first to resect and primarily reconstruct the obstructed ureteropelvic junction. In one article (*SC* 68) he mentioned fourteen such operations up to 1912.

When treating renal tuberculosis, the amount of parenchymal destruction was evaluated to determine whether to do nephrectomy or only pyeloplasty for obstruction (*SC* 228). He claimed that the tubercular kidney would heal, just as the lung would, with rest and supportive therapy. If nephrectomy was done, the cut end of ureter left behind was carefully inverted by a purse-string suture to discourage fistulization.

For renal abscesses he advocated surgical drainage as a first step and subcapsular nephrectomy several months later (*SC* 411).

He described well the renal anatomy, including the relationships to neighboring organs; he cautioned that kidney neoplasms should be handled gently to avoid spreading metastases; he was aware that flank pain is a late symptom of renal cancer.

PROSTATE

It is remarkable that even though vesical calculi had been treated by surgery for over two thousand years, the role of the enlarged prostate in causing bladder neck obstruction was not fully understood until the latter half of the nineteenth century, and its treatment by prostatectomy was not established until after the turn of the century.

George Goodfellow was credited with performing the first successful perineal prostatectomy in 1891, which was reported in 1904 in a series of 78 such operations (4, p. 393). The procedure was popularized by Hugh Hampton Young, and in the late nineteenth century the perineal approach was the preferred operation in the United States. It was not until sometime after Peter Freyer of Great Britain recommended the suprapubic approach in 1901 (1) that that path was accepted. Freyer subsequently reported 1,625 cases done suprapubically with a mortality of only 5 percent (2).

By the early 1900s, Murphy was teaching that repeated catheterization led to serious urinary tract infection and was advising prostatectomy to avoid this situation. In his usual manner, he reviewed the subject in depth in a monograph published in the *JAMA* in 1902 (JBM 60). In it he reported his first 8 patients. By 1916, he had done over 1,000 prostatectomies and reported that his mortality rates had fallen from 10 percent in the first 100 to 4.5 percent in the last 400 (*SC* 581, p. 939).

Freyer's extremely low mortality rate impressed Murphy but at first he was more influenced by H. H. Young. Therefore, in his earlier patients he generally used the perineal approach unless the obstruction was high in the gland, which was true about 25 percent of the time (JBM 63; 69; 81). Later, in 1912, he had reversed those figures, noting that "we are doing four of these operations by the suprapubic route to one by the perineal" (*SC* 57, p. 514). This was done because there was less risk of injury to the urethra.

For both approaches, Murphy preferred not to use a sound, and for the suprapubic approach, he inserted his left fore and middle fingers into the rectum to press the prostate forward to the enucleating right forefinger. After the perineal operation, he made no attempt to unite the bladder and urethral mucosa and simply left a catheter in place.

Before prostatectomy he advised vasectomy as a prophylaxis against postoperative epididymitis (*SC* 294, p. 1035). This was probably not his own innovation since vasectomy for this purpose had been recommended in 1906 by Prastin. Postoperatively, the bladder was kept free of clots with a syphonage system Murphy called Bremerman's apparatus, which was pictured in volume 581 of the *Surgical Clinics* (p. 937).

Murphy could not believe that a transurethral approach to prostatic obstruction would be satisfactory. When Bottini began making linear incisions into the gland transurethrally with a galvanocautery to produce a slough, Murphy used the instrument suprapubically instead (JBM 60). Even in 1916 in the *Surgical Clinics* (*SC* 581), he mentioned only the suprapubic and perineal approaches as options for prostatectomy.

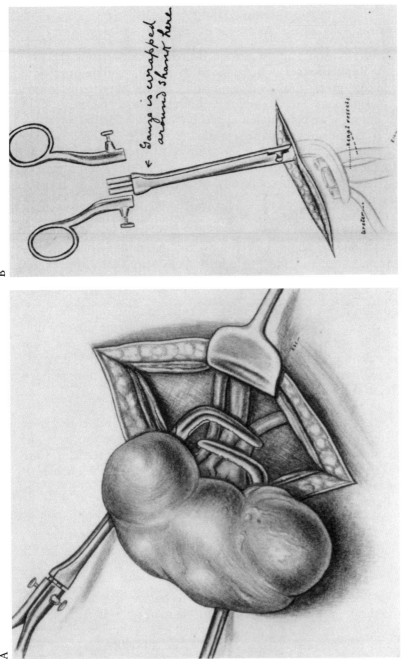

Fig. 8.1. Murphy's technique for nephrectomy. (A) The pedicle was not always clamped in toto. (B) When a clamp was left on the pedicle, the handles were detached and the shanks were tied with gauze. The wound was closed around the clamp.

BLADDER

Bladder stone was a common problem. In recommending his treatment, Murphy said that "a certain degree of risk attends the prolonged manipulations which are necessary in the crushing operation; we therefore prefer lithotomy, and advocate the suprapubic route. Until recent years lateral perineal lithotomy was the method of choice, but now we believe that approach to the bladder by this route entails an undue amount of unnecessary trauma" (*SC* 524).

The only bladder tumors mentioned by Murphy are papillomas. The smaller ones were removed transurethrally (*SC* 229), but large ones were attacked suprapubically with a combination of excision and cauterization (*SC* 391).

An operation he did for exstrophy of the bladder is intriguing (JBM 70). The patient was a twenty-year-old male who was incontinent since birth but for whom "erection, sexual desire and seminal emissions [were] normal." The physical findings were that "the penis is about 2 inches long. Glans well formed except defect in superior surface . . . the organ is curved upward and rests against the abdomen. The dorsum is open and the urethra is exposed. Just above the penis . . . is a bright red granular, eroded area protruding, the size of a dollar. . . . Between penis and this area are two small openings from which a clear amber urine trickles." In addition, there were diastasis recti, a separated symphasis pubis, inguinal hernias, and undescended testicles in inguinal folds.

In four operations the scar tissues were excised, the bladder was closed, the rectus muscles approximated, and the urethra closed over a catheter so that the urine was conducted into a rubber pouch. Nothing was done for the pubic separation or the hernias or testicles. Care was taken that "true skin was not inverted as it would put a hair-producing tissue in the bladder and therefore be fatal to the result, as phosphates and other salts would constantly form calculi."

Murphy estimated the constructed bladder capacity at only four to six cc. "I have a plan for the reestablishment of the sphincter vesicae internum and I feel it can be restored. Its nerve supply is still intact and only needs an approximation well unto the bladder wall to make it secure." There was no follow-up.

In view of Murphy's reluctance to recognize the value of the transurethral approach to the prostate, it is of interest that he was quite adept at cystoscopy and illustrated the technic with photographs in the *Surgical Clinics* (*SC* 229, pp. 345–48). He used this route to fulgurate bladder papillomas, but if they were too large he used the scope through a small cystotomy incision.

EXTERNAL GENITALIA

Murphy recommended conservative surgery for tuberculosis of the testicle. In a fifty-six-page article on the subject (JBM 57) he reviewed the disease and suggested that epididymectomy rather than orchiectomy should be used whenever possible (see also SC 309; 582). Paraffin prostheses were used to replace testicles resected for tuberculosis (SC 209) or for neoplasm (SC 355).

In contrast to today's thinking, he recommended bilateral orchiectomy for testicular tumors (SC 355) and he seemed willing to be quite radical in his surgical attack. While operating on a testicular tumor, he said, "I have asked for permission, in case this tumor turns out to be a sarcoma, to follow the excision of the testicle with an immediate laparotomy and dissect out all the retroperitoneal lymph-glands on the left side up as far as the kidney" (SC 310, p. 1201).

For undescended testes Murphy was content to mobilize them sufficiently to place them into the scrotum, which he first dilated, and to sew them to the bottom of the sac without further fixation to the thigh (SC 200; 437).

Among miscellaneous operations on the external genitalia Murphy reported: distal phallectomy and inguinal node resection for cancer of the penis (SC 283; 284); excision for urethral caruncle (SC 454; 578); plastic repair of a prolapse of a female urethra following trauma and previous surgery (SC 579); the Andrews "bottle" operation for hydrocele (SC 609); and varicocelectomy for scrotal discomfort and backache (SC 3).

TRAUMA

In an early but undated paper reprinted from the *Railway Surgeon* when he was the president of the National Association of Railway Surgeons and still a professor of surgery at the College of Physicians and Surgeons (somewhere between 1892 and 1895), Murphy reviewed "Traumatisms of the Urinary Tract" (JBM 4). For severe kidney injuries, blunt or penetrating, he recommended early operation to prevent shock from blood loss.

After bladder injuries in fractures of the pelvis, if the patient couldn't urinate, Murphy cautioned against forceful catheterization lest more damage be done. If a catheter could not be passed, a suprapubic extraperitoneal approach to the bladder was the first step and during it the bladder was to be opened and checked for rupture. Only if the upper bladder had a rent was the peritoneal cavity entered. Urethral injuries were repaired very early.

VACCINE THERAPY

In Chapter 10, Murphy's interest in vaccine treatment is reviewed, including a paper he and Kreuscher wrote on its use in diseases of the genitourinary tract (JBM 133). They were particularly concerned about "metastatic arthritides" that accompany urologic infections, and they included reports on five patients who were helped by vaccine even though three of them had recurrences that required retreatment. Their final conclusion was "that vaccines should always be used, but that up to the present time we are not justified in neglecting other known methods of combatting infections of the genitourinary tract and their sequelae."

REFERENCES

1. Freyer, P. J., "A clinical lecture on total extirpation of the prostate for radical cure of the enlargement of that organ," *British Medical Journal* 11 (1901): 125.

2. Freyer, P. J., *Clinical Lectures on Diseases of the Prostate,* 5th ed. (London: Bailliere, Tindoll, and Cox, 1920).

3. Gross, S. W., "Nephrectomy: Its indication and contraindication," *American Journal of Medical Sciences* 90 (1885): 79–90.

4. Murphy, L. J. I., *The History of Urology* (Springfield, Ill.: Thomas, 1972).

5. Raffensperger, J. G., personal communication, 1991.

9

VASCULAR SURGERY

Michael J. Verta and Robert L. Schmitz

In the 1890s John B. Murphy began working in his laboratory on blood vessel surgery and soon applied his work to trauma patients at Cook County Hospital. His papers on vascular surgery demonstrate his usual broad interest in all aspects of a field.

ARTERIAL SUTURE

Murphy did much experimental surgery on arteries in his search for a satisfactory technique for end-to-end anastomosis. Ultimately, he was content that he had a good method (*SC* 319) (fig. 9.1). This work was reported at the meeting of the International Medical Congress in Moscow in 1897 and was recorded in an article that was printed in three places (JBM 43; 48; 49).

He apparently applied his work in several patients, but the number is difficult to assess. In the articles describing his arterial experiments he mentioned two instances, one in which the femoral artery was ligated, not anastomosed (the patient recovered well), and the other in which the proximal femoral artery was invaginated into the distal vessel after resecting one-half inch of an injured part; four days after the latter operation there was a dorsalis pedis pulse in that limb and the patient was discharged some three months later with no edema and "no disturbance of circulation."

There were apparently some real end-to-end unions, however. In his report on the extraction of an iliac embolus (JBM 109) he stated that "the suture of an incision in an artery is as simple as the suture of an intestine, if a sufficiently small needle be used. This I demonstrated in 1896, at which time I made the first successful end-to-end union of an artery that had ever been made, excising half an inch of the femoral artery at about the same point where I incised today." Later in the article he wrote, "Since 1896 I have had two additional end-to-end sutures of arteries, one of the femoral in Scarpa's triangle for a bullet wound, and another of the first portion of the axillary just below the clavicle. In both, end-to-end union was effected by my suture method and the circulation in the extremity promptly restored. A little over five years later all three of these end-to-end unions were examined by Dr. Neff and the circulation in the extremities was found perfect." Murphy referred to these cases again (*SC* 190, p. 913) and added that "some of the men who are writing now have overlooked these cases." These quotations are of great importance in view of the controversy that exists over who did the first end-to-end arterial anastomosis.

Further on in the same article (JBM 109), he mentioned another remarkable operation, noting that "in September, 1908, a successful end-to-end anastomosis was made of the femoral artery into the femoral vein for endarteritis obliterans."

Finally, he wrote, "Since I published my original experiments and results in this line and demonstrated the feasibility of this work, Payr, Hoeffer, Exner, Ullman, Carrel, Guthrie and others have supported the practicability of arterial suture and demonstrated that extremities and organs can be transplanted and the circulation maintained." He was implying that his work antedated Carrel's, which appeared in the literature from 1902 to 1908 and earned the Nobel Prize in 1912. He made his claim to priority even clearer (*SC* 319, p. 72) when he said, "Carrel, when he was here in Chicago, took up with Guthrie the work of vascular suture where we left off." And then, of Carrel's organ transplant work he said, "Of course, such transplants will not functionate, because a transplanted organ, in order to live and functionate, must be not only from the same species, but also from the same individual." There are those who feel that some of Murphy's, as well as Carrel's, concepts came from Jaboulay's earlier work, but in spite of many references to the literature Murphy never mentions him or his work.

Matas and Bergan and Yao agree that Murphy's work has priority. Rudolph Matas in a paper given before the American Surgical Association (2) said, "Dorfler, Lindner, Israel, Salomoni, Tomaselli, Carrel and others . . . following in the wake of Murphy in arteriorraphy, have conclusively shown that the through-and-through suture of the arterial wall is not followed by thrombosis." (Note the position of Carrel's name in the quotation.) Bergan and Yao in their *Techniques in Arterial Surgery,* written in 1989, also give Murphy credit for "the first end-to-end suture of a human artery" (1).

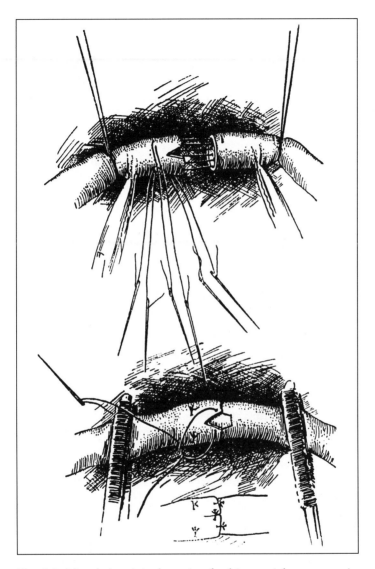

Fig. 9.1. Murphy's original caption for his arterial anastomosis:
The upper drawing shows one method of controlling the hemorrhage and steadying the vessel ends by ligatures gently tied; and
also the method of inserting the three double-needled mattress invaginating sutures. The lower drawing represents the vessels compressed by rubber-covered vessel clamps, the invaginating sutures
tied, and the approximation mattress suture being inserted. The
outline drawing shows all sutures tied.

ANEURYSM

Murphy did animal experimental work on repairing aneurysms and devised his own method of endoaneurysmorraphy, which he reported at a New Orleans meeting of the American Medical Association. This work, however, was apparently not published, perhaps because, as Murphy admitted, "I think Matas' suture method is better than the plan I had advocated previously" (*SC* 319, p. 66).

Murphy recorded an operation on a false aneurysm on a syphilitic axillary artery that had caused brachial plexus paralysis by pressure (*SC* 190). He first gained proximal control by dividing the clavicle and passing a ligature around the subclavian artery. He solved the local problem by ligating the axillary artery above and below the aneurysm and relied on the collateral circulation to supply the arm. The patient gained excellent recovery of muscular function.

While operating on an endarteritic aneurysm of the brachial artery in the mid-arm (*SC* 319), he gave a magnificent overview of aneurysmal disease, including histology, etiology, classification (for which he presented a list), and treatment. At the operation, he did a Matas endoaneurysmorraphy. For temporary arterial occlusion during the surgery Murphy used "little spring forceps . . . used commonly in operations on the muscles of the eye."

CERVICAL RIB

In 1904 (JBM 86), Murphy saw a patient who had had tingling in the index and little fingers of the left hand on and off for a year and a half. The left forearm and hand were always cold. On examination, Murphy could feel a rib in the neck that seemed to arise from the seventh cervical vertebra. When pain developed in the wrist and thumb, operation was advised. The entire rib was excised, and the patient was totally relieved of his symptoms.

In 1906 (JBM 96), Murphy saw a patient with a goiter who also had a stinging pain down the arm to the hand and fingers when pressure was applied over a hard mass in the right supraclavicular fossa. An X-ray examination showed a cervical rib on the right. In two separate operations Murphy removed first the goiter and then the rib. The arm symptoms were relieved.

There are accounts of three more operations for cervical ribs in the *Surgical Clinics* (*SC* 45; 427; 476). In the last one, he gave a complete overview using a collective review of 112 references by Darling. He described two distinct sets of symptoms, those from arterial pressure and those from brachial plexus pressure. He recommended an incision along the anterior border of the scalenus anticus muscle and suggested taking the rib out from the base forward.

While Murphy contributed nothing original to the treatment of cervical ribs, his operations were done relatively early in the surgical approach to this problem.

VARICOSE VEINS

Murphy presented "A Talk on Varicose Veins and Varicose Leg Ulcers" (*SC* 558), in which he said it was "an old and hackneyed subject, still they form a large percentage of one's practice, and the mere fact that so much is constantly being written about them goes to show that there are many knotty problems." He then offered one of his extensive overviews of the problem and its various recommended operations. Later in the *Clinics* (*SC* 585) he recorded multiple resections in the thigh and leg for varices.

Commenting on the cicatricial scars produced by some vein operations (*SC* 397), he cautioned against the Schede operation in which "a complete annular division of the skin around the leg, including the veins" was made below the knee, and he cited two cases in which the scar contracture led to gangrene, of half the foot in one and of one toe in the other.

Because he found the usual "clam-shell cast" used in the treatment of stasis ulcers clumsy and difficult to apply, he devised a lace-on "leg corset" of heavy-grade linen or silk from the ankle to the head of the tibia (JBM 107). He also used it to relieve the "leg fatigue" that accompanies varicose veins even when they have not ulcerated. It is of interest that in the 1940s and 1950s a version of this legging containing an inflatable rubber bladder to exert even pressure was advocated by W. J. Merle Scott of the University of Rochester School of Medicine, New York (3).

COMMON ILIAC EMBOLISM

Murphy reported a remarkable operation for removal of an embolus from the common iliac artery (JBM 109). The patient, a forty-one-year-old woman, presented with pain in the left lower chest and upper abdomen that disappeared when the pain shifted to her pelvis and legs. At first both legs became cold but the right one warmed up while the left one became blue from the thigh down and blebs began to appear. It wasn't until the fourth day of the illness that Murphy saw the patient when she was admitted to Mercy Hospital. He took her to the operating room immediately.

"Nitrous oxide was given for thirty seconds, while an incision four inches long was made downward from an inch above Poupart's ligament to the femoral artery. . . . The anesthesia was then stopped . . . and the femoral artery was exposed for a distance of 2 1/2 inches." An incision one-inch long was made in the artery, which was found to be completely thrombosed. "With a delicate forceps the clot (a bifurcated plug an inch and a half long) was drawn from below upward, when fresh arterial blood came from below. . . ." Cleaning out the proximal clot proved more difficult but Murphy persisted with forceps, spoons, various catheters, and finally a uterine sound until an "intense arterial flow, carrying with it a lot of embolic debris and fresh, bright blood" was obtained.

"At the line of demarcation the circulation was improved immediately . . . becoming well marked a considerable distance lower." Later an amputation was done in the lower leg and the flap survived.

In his summation of this experience and his experimental work on thrombi, he suggested that even cerebral ischemia from emboli lodged in the common or internal carotid arteries should be amenable to extraction. He suggested that aspiration through a catheter would probably be the best technic and that any incision used for extraction should be made away from the area of the thrombus to minimize rethrombosis, so apt to occur at the point where the original plug had lodged.

The evidence seems to support Murphy's claim that he did the first successful end-to-end arterial anastomosis in man. His attack on a common iliac embolus would be appropriate even today.

REFERENCES

1. Bergan, J. J., and J. S. T. Yao, *Techniques in Arterial Surgery* (Philadelphia: Saunders, 1989), 5.

2. Ravitch, M. M., *A Century of Surgery* (Philadelphia: Lippincott, 1981), vol. 1, p. 342.

3. Scott, W. J. M., "Postphlebitic and varicose venous stasis; clinical results of treatment by pulsatile air-pressure principle," *JAMA* 147 (1950): 1195–1201.

10

INFECTIOUS DISEASES

Warren W. Furey and Robert L. Schmitz

Although his focus was on surgery, Murphy had considerable experience with some infectious diseases. He included them in his writings seemingly in the sequence in which he encountered them.

ACTINOMYCOSIS

His very first publication (JBM 1) dealt with actinomycosis. It was a paper he read before the Chicago Medical Society on December 15, 1884, in which he summarized the literature dealing with the disease (there were twenty-eight instances) and presented two patients of his own.

The first patient was a twenty-eight-year-old female who had had a toothache two weeks earlier in the lower jaw, followed by swelling in the throat, dysphagia, and trismus. When Murphy saw the patient, the left tonsil filled the pharynx and was pointing. He opened the abscess and released a large quantity of creamy pus. The patient did well for a while but then a mass the size of a walnut appeared in the left neck. Incision yielded creamy pus that contained sulphur-colored granules on microscopic examination which were considered to be actinomycetes.

With the assistance of Drs. Fenger, Belfield, and Verity, Murphy excised and debrided the left neck and extracted a carious tooth after which a probe passed readily through the alveolus into the neck wound. A bit of the mandible was removed and the alveolus was curetted. A tampon was placed in the alveolus, the neck was drained, and the wound was closed with silk. Primary union occurred and the patient gained twenty-six pounds in five weeks.

The second patient was an eighteen-year-old male who had had a toothache for two months when a pigeon-egg-sized swelling appeared below the jaw near the tooth. Puncturing of the mass yielded a small amount of thick, creamy pus that on microscopic examination contained "typical" actinomycetes. The incised mass was scraped on two occasions but Murphy did not comment on the final outcome.

In a second paper, read before the Chicago Medical Society on October 5, 1891 (JBM 11), he reviewed the history of actinomycosis. It was not recognized as an entity until 1877 when Bollinger described it as a disease of cattle. Later the same year, Israel described two instances in man but did not realize it was the same disease Bollinger had reported. It was Porifick, in 1879, who suggested that the disease was the same in both species.

By this time Murphy had treated five patients, four with jaw involvement, all of whom recovered, and one with abdominal disease who died. He suggested that the treatment should be radical extirpation, the dissection to be guided by the characteristic golden yellow slough. He felt that those lesions that could not be surgically removed would end fatally.

TUBERCULOSIS

During his "wandering year" in Europe, Murphy had an episode of hematuria that was interpreted to be renal tuberculosis. The diagnosis seemed logical since two brothers, David and Frank, and a sister, Lucinda, died of pulmonary tuberculosis. Later in his life he developed a "pulmonary problem" that was also considered to be tubercular and he spent eight months recuperating in Colorado Springs, Colorado, and in Las Vegas, Nevada. (It is interesting that at his autopsy no evidence of tuberculosis was found.)

With this background it is natural that he developed a considerable interest in tuberculosis; many of his articles and his *Surgical Clinics* reports dealt with this disease and many of his letters were to tubercular patients he sent to Colorado Springs to recuperate.

Tuberculosis was one of the most common causes of death in Murphy's era and he devoted many pages to it in his large monograph *Surgery of the Lung* (JBM 54), published in 1898 (see Chapter 7). Murphy quoted an autopsy series in which there was evidence of tuberculous lesions either active or healed in over 75 percent of patients dying suddenly of other causes. He stated that the evidence of repaired tuberculosis in the lung was so common the Germans had an axiom that every man by the time of death had had at least a little tuberculosis.

One of Murphy's earliest attempts at treating this disease was reported in one of his first articles (JBM 8), entitled "Observations on the Use of Koch Lymph with Report of Eleven Cases." He reviewed in depth what was known about the lymph (tuberculin), and listed the general reactions of chills, fever, pain in the limbs, coughing, fatigue, and vomiting, and the local reactions of swelling and redness. He then described in detail, often with temperature charts, eleven patients he had treated. In six the disease was in bone or joint; in one, in nodes; and in four, in the lungs. They were started on one mg of Koch lymph and the dose increased one mg per day until a "reaction was obtained." Murphy wrote, "These cases are reported for the purpose of demonstrating that there is a specific reaction produced by the remedy, the question of permanent cure being left for the future." In four of them, he said, "we feel that the injections had a curative effect."

Studies of repaired tuberculosis of the lung had shown cicatrization of lung tissue, greatly thickened pleura, and contraction of the chest wall so that the motion of the diseased lung was restricted, that is, the body had promoted healing of the diseased part by putting it at rest. But the bony ribcage often prevented pulmonary cavities from collapsing and thereby interfered with healing. This chest-wall rigidity could be overcome by operations such as Shede's, which removed the ribs and allowed the cavities to collapse, empty through the bronchus, and heal by obliteration.

Murphy was aware of cases of tuberculous hydrothorax in which there was complete recovery of the lung. He reasoned that compression of the lung by the fluid, with resultant quiescence and collapse of cavities, favored healing.

In his 1898 oration he described five patients in whom he injected sterile nitrogen into the pleural space to compress the lung (JBM 54, p. 341) (see Chapter 7) and gave the exact technic and amount of the gas to be used. Three other attempts were not successful because the presence of adhesions prevented lung collapse. He believed this technic to be best suited for patients with apical or monolobar tuberculosis in the early stages. He reinjected one patient and thought this might be necessary in other patients, at six- to ten-week intervals or as indicated. To save time, he turned over to his associate, August F. Lemke, the administration of pneumothorax, and by 1914 some 460 patients had been given some 2,000 pneumothoracies.

Before the Chicago Medical Society on January 7, 1914, at a symposium on tuberculosis (JBM 131), Murphy seemed to disregard his prepared paper and gave instead a very comprehensive overview of the disease that included comparative pathology of avian versus bovine infection, portals of entry, susceptibility of various tissues, the histology of local lesions and local resistance, the importance of rest in treatment, the role of opsonins, the methods of diagnosis, tuberculin in diagnosis and treatment, and finally the value of pneumothorax. It was a truly magnificent ad lib presentation.

In addition to the pulmonary variety, Murphy treated patients with tuberculosis in the bones, joints, genitalia, urinary tract, and gastrointestinal tract. These sites are covered in the appropriate chapters.

TYPHOID

In 1903, Murphy discussed general peritonitis and its high mortality rate (JBM 71). He described six patients who had perforation of the gastrointestinal tract, five from appendicitis and one from typhoid of the terminal ileum.

The last patient was thirty-five years old and in the third week of an attack of typhoid fever when he experienced sudden sharp pain paraumbilically. The pain became generalized; distention and vomiting developed. Murphy first saw him at home and immediately placed him in a semi-sitting position. There was tympany over the upper abdomen and dullness in the right lower abdomen. The patient was kept in the same position during the transfer to the hospital, during the operation, and postoperatively.

At operation, about seven hours after the onset of pain, a 4.5 mm perforation was found in the ileum 14 cm from the ileocecal valve at the center of an indurated Peyer's patch. The perforation was sutured shut and two half-inch drains were placed into the pelvis and brought out at the lower angle of the incision. These drains were irrigated with normal saline solution, saline proctoclysis was administered, and a streptococcal vaccine was injected. The patient was discharged twenty-four days later. The five patients with appendiceal rupture were handled in much the same manner and all recovered.

In a later paper, in 1915 (JBM 138), Murphy discussed the plight of a sixteen-year-old lad admitted to the hospital with fever and acute sharp and shooting pain in the lumbar region radiating to the abdomen. There were no chills, nausea, or vomiting. The attacks lasted thirty to sixty minutes and came two hours after mealtime. From the history Murphy learned that the boy had had typhoid fever five months before. He made a diagnosis of typhoid spondylitis. A plaster jacket was applied extending from the arms to the hips and the patient was confined to bed. The pain decreased and the temperature fell to normal. The Widal was positive, but of greater importance, bacillus typhosus was isolated from a blood culture. The boy was "therefore a typhoid carrier."

Murphy wrote, "We know the common lurking places of the typhoid bacilli are the gallbladder and the appendix so that is why the appendix will be removed and the gallbladder drained. He is a source of danger to himself by developing a metastatic infection in the vertebral joint but he menaces his community by scattering typhoid bacilli. We know it is difficult to get rid of the bacillus typhosus. We will also prepare a vaccine from autogenous cultures from the bile grown on his own red blood cells."

Murphy then proceeded to do an appendectomy and to drain the gallbladder. Cultures of bile and the appendix teemed with bacillus typhosus. Cultures of stool, urine, and bile eventually became free of bacilli, the gallbladder drainage tube was removed, and the patient was sent home—all this without antibiotics.

The spondylitis "without caries" is probably the same type of arthropathy we see associated with Salmonellal disease and the B17 genotype that is so difficult to explain precisely. Murphy was especially pleased that this was the first time the carrier state had been recognized by first diagnosing typhoid spondylitis.

TETANUS

That Murphy was a bold, self-confident man is brought out in his treatment of a youth with tetanus (JBM 82). The patient was eight years old and was admitted to Mercy Hospital on July 10, 1904. He had stepped on glass seven days previously. The wound had been washed and an antiphlogistin applied, which had been prescribed by a physician who had not seen the boy. Six days after the accident stiffness of the jaws was noted followed in twenty-four hours by trismus and spasms of the muscles of the neck and back. There were no chills, fever, or sweats. There was little inflammation about the wound.

On the boy's admission to the hospital, the trismus was pronounced and every three to five minutes there was contraction of the muscles of the back and neck with marked opisthotonus. The patient was anesthetized, the wounds were opened, curetted, cauterized, and packed with iodoform gauze. Glass and some pus were encountered. When the patient awakened, convulsions came every ten to fifteen minutes and lasted one to three minutes. Temperature was 99.8 degrees and pulse was 110. On July 11 he was given three full doses of antitetanic serum without effect. Convulsions became almost continuous.

On the morning of July 13 a lumbar puncture was made and 16 cc of a cloudy cerebrospinal fluid were withdrawn and at the same time 3 cc of the following solution were injected into the subarachnoid space:

Rx	B. eucain gr.iss	09
	Morphin sulphate gr. 1/3	02
	Sodium chloridi gr. iii	18
	Distilled water ozs.iiiss	105

This solution had been sterilized by boiling. The patient slept four hours following the injection and through the night slept an hour and a half at a time. The spasms became of shorter duration and he had only eight in the next twenty-four hours. When spasms recurred he received retreatments on July 14, 15, and 16; on July 17 no treatment was given because he seemed better. He could now talk well and get a good night's rest. He had three more treatments on July 19, 20, and 21. Following this he had no more spasm and the trismus cleared. He was discharged on July 31.

Murphy felt many tetanus patients died from exhaustion from the severity of the spasms, including those of the respiratory muscles. He felt these could be overcome with intrathecal injections such as he used in this patient and next time he planned to increase the dose of eucain to one-sixth or one-third grain with each injection. Murphy also felt that repeated spinal punctures relieved spinal fluid pressure and gave the greatest percentage of recoveries.

Encouraged by the success in this patient, Murphy wrote (JBM 82) that he saw

> no reason why the cerebrospinal cavities cannot be washed out in severe infections with salt or other neutralizing solutions by the following method, which I plan to put into practice in the first case of meningitis coming under my observation: first, make a drill puncture of the cranium over the lateral ventricle; insert a fine needle until the C.S.F. escapes; second, insert a needle into the spinal canal in the lumbar region and allow a normal salt solution to drip under hydrostatic pressure from the needle in the lateral ventricle, down through the foramen of Magendie and the spinal canal to and out of the needle in the lumbar area. This can be accomplished on the cadaver as I have demonstrated.

However, he did not publish on either tetanus or the "Murphy wash" for meningitis again. Nevertheless, this method has been subsequently used by others.

SYPHILIS

In 1910 Murphy discussed (JBM 112) the Ehrlich-Hata preparation known as 606 or salvarsan, diamidoarsenobenzol dihydrochloride, "a single injection of which is reported to be destructive of the Spirochaeta pallida; this arsenical is thought to be as destructive of spirochetes as quinine is of the plasmodia of malaria."

His information was apparently second hand from Dr. C. H. McKenna of Chicago who was in Paris when Murphy asked him to go to Frankfurt to see Professor Ehrlich. McKenna was received with the greatest courtesy and "all matters concerning this preparation, the treatment and results were placed at his disposal for observation." Over an eleven-month period seven thousand patients had been treated; Professor Ehrlich considered that only one of six deaths might be related to treatment. The drug seemed to have the specific property of killing spirochetes in all its abodes in tissue, in all three stages of the disease—primary, secondary, and tertiary.

On the basis of these second-hand reports Murphy opines, "regardless of what its permanent effect in definitely curing syphilis by a single dose may be, its immediate effect places it far beyond any medicament that has been so far used in the treatment of this disease and makes one feel that every sufferer should have the advantage that it affords."

At the end of the article, Murphy said he was awaiting a special supply of twenty-five doses of 606 that Professor Ehrlich kindly was providing through Dr. McKenna. Murphy planned to compare its effectiveness with that of sodium cacodylate, but there are no reports of such comparative studies.

Then, in 1912, he counters, "Salvarsan has not fulfilled its expectations. It was supposed and believed by those who advocated its early use that one injection would bring about a cure. That is already entirely out of consideration" (*SC* 5, p. 32). To improve its effectiveness, Murphy was repeating the injections every three weeks until the Wassermann became negative. He was also adding injections of bichlorid of mercury and sodium cacodylate hypodermically but not intravenously since there had been some deaths from the latter route.

Finally in 1914 Murphy concluded that "with sodium cacodylate chancres heal in 6 or 7 days, much faster than with 606" (*SC* 363).

Sodium cacodylate had already been used by him for seven years "to relieve the pain of metastatic osseous carcinoma." He now employed this drug alone in the treatment of syphilis and reported "clearing of spirochetes" in forty-eight hours from mucous patches and primary chancres.

Interestingly, cost was also an influencing factor in Murphy's preference for sodium cacodylate, as salvarsan listed at thirty to thirty-five dollars an ounce. He said, "I think sodium cacodylate is the therapeutic agent of the future. Fifteen cents' worth is sufficient to cure a chancre."

Murphy continued, "If we can cure the primary lesion in 6, 8 or 10 days, the syphilis problem is mastered. Why? Because the danger of transmission is thereby minimized. It is from the primary and secondary manifestations and discharges that contagion occurs." At this stage Murphy seemed to recognize that the arsenicals might not be curative, but they at least made an infected individual unlikely to transmit the disease.

Murphy was publishing "these incomplete reports . . . merely as suggestions to practitioners who are willing to try a remedy as safe as sodium cacodylate and who have numerous cases coming under their observation, as the only syphilitic cases I encounter are those presenting as surgical lesions. I would further suggest the primary dose be from 2 to 4 grains depending on size and strength of the patient and not be repeated within 3 or 4 days unless there are specific indications."

Murphy's other discussions of syphilis were mostly concerning Charcot joints and their surgical management and are found in the *Surgical Clinics*. He prided himself on making diagnoses of Charcot joints others had missed because of the absence of pain.

ECHINOCOCCUS

There is a single mention of echinococcus disease among Murphy's papers. It appears in one titled only "Surgical Clinic" (JBM 12). He had been invited to present a talk before the Chicago Medical Society at Cook County Hospital. He had Dr. Sippy, the house surgeon, present the history and then had two students from Rush Medical College, La Count and Bishop, examine the patient. (These men all became prominent in the field of medicine.) It developed that the patient had an echinococcus cyst of the liver that had been proven by earlier aspiration.

He quizzed the students and by this approach drew out the essentials of the life cycle, pathology, diagnosis, and treatment of the disease. He recommended Langenbach's two-stage operation and that was how he had already treated this patient. First, a transperitoneal operation was done to stimulate adhesions between the liver and the parietal peritoneum. At the next stage the cyst in the liver was marsupialized by cutting into the liver through the lower chest wall, transpleurally, by cautery. Then the wound was dressed until the cyst had been obliterated.

At the end of the presentation, he thanked each student by name, saying, "I must compliment you on your excellent answers, and the thorough knowledge which you have shown on the subject, and in doing so, I am sure I am only expressing the sentiment of the members of the Society, as you have not been prompted and have not seen the case previous to its presentation here tonight."

VACCINES

In a *Surgical Clinics* report (*SC* 154), Philip Kreuscher presented the work he and Murphy had done on the preparation and therapeutic use of auto-vaccines. The details of preparation of auto-vaccines were spelled out and then their use was described in a wide variety of infections that were referred to the two doctors for surgical therapy "as a last resort": acne vulgaris, furuncles, carbuncles, glandular infections (not tubercular), asthma and hay fever, empyema, persistent draining wounds scattered over the body, and genitourinary infections.

Kreuscher and Murphy became particularly interested in the metastatic arthritides, which they felt followed infections elsewhere in the body, e.g., tonsils, sinuses, dental, and genito-urinary tract. In a paper read after Murphy's death (JBM 141), Kreuscher said that "in the last three years we have devoted our best efforts to the vaccine treatment of acute and chronic joint infections (arthritis)" and described an experience with ninety cases.

They distinguished three classes of arthritis patients: 1) "That type of deforming arthritis of gradual and insidious onset from which no organism can be obtained, either from the joints or blood streams, nor from the secretions or excretions"; 2) "Those cases, mostly of the chronic variety, which had their origin in ancient infection of the mouth, pharynx, tonsils, respiratory tract, intestinal tract, from which we were unable to obtain any one specific organism at the time the patients came for treatment, but who yielded to mixed vaccines"; 3) "Those patients with acute or chronic infections of the joints in which we are able to isolate a distinct organism or organisms which we believe to have been the cause of the trouble." Reports of favorable outcomes were presented but no overall numbers or estimates of the percentage of responders were given.

In another paper (JBM 133), "Vaccine Treatment of Diseases of the Genito-Urinary Tract," the method of preparation was again outlined and a footnote described a modification suggested by Murphy to improve their vaccines by growing "the culture for autogenous vaccines upon media which are wholly or partially made up of the patient's own blood. . . . A detailed report . . . will be published at a later date." It never was.

"In summing up our experience with vaccine therapy of genito-urinary infections, and the sequelae, especially the metastatic arthridites, covering a series of not less than 100 cases" (only six cured patients are presented), the authors drew these conclusions:

1. That autogenous vaccines should be used in all cases when it is possible to obtain them, but that there are cases in which there is a positive indication for combined vaccines.

2. That vaccines have failed in many instances because of the insurmountable difficulties in obtaining the proper organisms from the genito-urinary tract and from insufficient drainage of the infected areas.

3. That vaccines must not be expected to reconstruct tissues, organs or joints that have been destroyed by known or unknown pathogenic organisms. That they are prophylactic against such destruction, and to be effective must be timely and intelligently administered.

4. That vaccines should always be used, but that up to the present time we are not justified in neglecting other known methods of combatting infections of the genito-urinary tract and their sequelae.

It is remarkable that Murphy, so busy and so involved with the avant-garde aspects of surgery, could have had as much experience as he did with the almost purely medical discipline of infectious disease. He even had time for some very basic work in this area.

11

AN APPRAISAL

Robert L. Schmitz

While Murphy may have been disliked by some and may have had his detractors, the national and international leaders in medicine and surgery seem to have considered him a genius. Our review of the details of his practice bears out this impression.

He was one of the pioneers who made surgery a specialty. While there were not yet Specialty Board requirements, he had his own standards for who should do surgery and he railed against the untrained "pseudo-surgeon" (Chapter 2).

Murphy emphasized the importance of the experimental laboratory in furthering the surgeon's skill and surgical science. He routinely tested new ideas and procedures in his animal operating room and it was there he worked out the details of the button, blood vessel anastomosis, peripheral nerve repair, bone grafting, arthroplasty, and how to overcome open pneumothorax, among other issues.

His skills in physical examination were great (Chapter 2) and some of the maneuvers he invented are still used and carry his eponym. Murphy's diagnostic acumen and surgical ability in the fields of general, gynecologic, neurologic, orthopedic, thoracic, urologic, and vascular surgery have been enumerated in the appropriate chapters of this book and are truly awesome.

He did the first operation for "early" appendicitis. To overcome formidable resistance to this concept, he followed and reported at frequent intervals on two thousand of his own appendectomies to establish that early operation was the safest treatment with the lowest mortality for acute appendicitis.

The Murphy button made digestive tract anastomosis possible at an earlier date and led to the development of proper suture technics for intestinal and biliary surgery. The principles of the button are the basis for present-day stapling instruments wherever used: gastrointestinal tract, genitourinary tract, biliary tract, or blood vessels. Various modifications of the button are still being used and new variations are still being devised.

Other pioneering work can be attributed to Murphy. His early work on blood vessel anastomosis opened the field. His delineation and utilization of the blood supply around joints in his arthroplasties presaged the present-day multi-tissue grafts based on regional blood supply. His advocacy of pneumothorax for pulmonary tuberculosis was important in establishing its value, whether or not he did it first. Until appropriate drugs came on the scene, this procedure was the mainstay of tuberculotherapy.

His methods of treating peritonitis and ileus led the way for marked improvement in the mortality and morbidity of these maladies. He stressed the need to diagnose mechanical intestinal obstruction accurately and to interfere surgically early in its course. The Murphy Drip for hydration of patients with ileus and/or peritonitis heralded principles that are still used for patient support. Murphy was an early user of chemotherapy and diagnostic and therapeutic radiology.

The *Surgical Clinics of North America* in large part owes its existence to him. Along with Franklin Martin, Murphy was a founder of the journal *Surgery, Gynecology and Obstetrics,* and he later became its editor.

He was a founder of and an active participant in the American College of Surgeons, the first body to try to regulate hospital quality and the ethical behavior of surgeons.

George Crile felt that "the place of America in Surgery is due more to the brilliant discoveries of Murphy and their forceful presentation than to the work of any other American; and he taught the world what it knows about abdominal surgery and the surgery of tuberculosis, the blood vessels and bone and joints" (*SC* 591, p. 993).

All in all, Murphy emerges as a brilliant thinker, an enthusiastic teacher, an avid experimenter, an accomplished, technically superb surgeon, and an unbelievably productive individual who kept abreast of surgical progress on an international scope.

THE BIBLIOGRAPHY OF JOHN B. MURPHY

Robert L. Schmitz and Timothy T. Oh

In attempting to catalogue our Murphy material we could not find an adequate bibliography of his writings. Since his publications are many and often very detailed, it seemed essential to compile as complete a listing as possible if we wished to evaluate his contributions.

The task was not an easy one. The listings in the *Index Medicus* use only initials for the first and middle names of authors, and we discovered two other J. B. Murphys, James and Joseph, whose articles we had to identify in order to eliminate them. An error in this regard is found in I. M. Rutkow's "A History of the Surgical Clinics of North America" (*SC* 67:1238), where reference 18 gives credit to John B. Murphy for a paper actually written by Fred B. Murphy of St. Louis.

The reprints in Murphy's files were usually just that: reprintings in monograph form starting with page one rather than the actual journal page number. We have about fifty such reprints in our collection and had to seek out the originals to list the correct page numbers. We discovered also that we have reprints that are not listed in the *Index Medicus*: JBM 4; 7; 10; 23; 34.

Many of Murphy's papers are duplicates, since he was frequently invited to speak and the societies he addressed often had their own periodicals in which his presentations were then printed. Of necessity, the same paper was read more than once and thus might be published as often as three or four times. Many of the monographs are of small-book length and required three or four issues of a periodical to be published. Since they were presented at society meetings, one wonders if an audience sat through an entire paper.

The currents of Murphy's major interests run through the journal articles. Tuberculosis appears very early and occurs throughout while orthopedics appears relatively late and dominates the later years. Appendicitis, the anastomotic button, and gallbladder disease are clustered between 1892 and 1897 while urological diseases and peritonitis appear later. The neurosurgical entries are three clusters representing trigeminal neuralgia, spinal cord lesions, and peripheral nerve trauma, in that order. The single thoracic paper is a large monograph covering the entire field up to that time.

As we have noted earlier, Murphy lectured continuously while he was operating; his remarks were taken down by a secretary for the hospital record and included much more than the report of the operation. His visitors began to request copies of these notes, so he hired an assistant, Margaret Maloney, for the purpose of assembling the notes for distribution. The demand became so great that Murphy negotiated with W. B. Saunders Company of Philadelphia to print the records in book form, and thus was born *The Surgical Clinics of John B. Murphy, M.D., at Mercy Hospital, Chicago.* The first edition appeared in February 1912 and the books have continued ever since. In 1914 the title was shortened by dropping the word *Surgical;* in 1917 it became *The Surgical Clinics of Chicago;* and in 1921 the present title, *Surgical Clinics of North America,* was adopted.

Books and Book Chapters

1. *General Surgery.* Chicago: Year Book Publishers, 1901–16. Murphy was the sole author in 1901–2 and was the editor during 1903–16.
2. "Intestinal Surgery." In *Gynecology and Abdominal Surgery,* ed. H. A. Kelly. Philadelphia and London: Saunders, 1908.
3. "Procedentia Uteri and the Appendix." In *Surgery: Its Principles and Practice,* ed. W. W. Keen. Philadelphia and London: Saunders, 1906–16.
4. *The Surgical Clinics of John B. Murphy, M.D., at Mercy Hospital in Chicago,* vols. 1–2; *The Clinics of John B. Murphy, M.D., at Mercy Hospital in Chicago,* vols. 3–5. Philadelphia and London: Saunders, 1912–16.

Journal Articles

1. "Actinomycosis in the human subject." *New York Medical Journal* 41 (1885): 17–19.
2. "Tubercular arthritis of the knee-joint, with excision." *Polyclinic* 5 (1887–88): 164.
3. "Gunshot wounds of the abdomen." *Chicago Medical Journal and Examiner* 56 (1888): 129–34.
4. "Traumatisms of the urinary tract." *Railway Surgeon* 2 (1895–96): 145–57.
5. "Tubercular arthritis of the knee-joint, with excision." *Medical Age* 7 (1889): 411–13.
6. "Early treatment of perityphlitis." *Western Medical Reporter* 11 (1889): 282–91.
7. "On early operation in perityphlitis" [coauthored with E. W. Lee]. No journal title given (1890).
8. "Observations on the use of the Koch lymph with report of eleven cases" [coauthored with E. W. Lee]. *Medical and Surgical Report of Cook County Hospital, 1890* (1891): 85–104.
9. "Observations on the use of the Koch lymph with report of eleven cases" [coauthored with E. W. Lee]. *North American Practitioner* 3 (1891): 193–207.

10. "Actinomycosis hominis, with report of five cases." *North American Practitioner* 3 (1891): 593–607.

11. "Actinomycosis hominis, with report of five cases." *Chicago Medical Record* 2 (1891–92): 485–99.

12. "Surgical clinic." *Chicago Medical Record*. April 1892.

13. "Two cases of appendicitis in contrast." *Chicago Clinical Review* 1 (1892–93): 116–18.

14. "A contribution to abdominal surgery; ideal approximation of abdominal viscera without suture." *North American Practitioner* 4 (1892): 481–98.

15. "Cholecysto-intestinal, gastro-intestinal, entero-intestinal anastomosis and approximation without sutures (original research)." *Medical Record* 42 (1892): 665–76.

16. "Some remarks on appendicitis, based upon one hundred and ten laparotomies and experimental investigations." *Kansas City Medical Index* 15 (1894): 40–42.

17. "Operative surgery of the gall-tracts, with original report of seventeen successful cholecystenterostomies by means of the anastomosis button." *Medical Record* 45 (1894) 35–42, 68–72.

18. "Operative surgery of the gall tracts, with original report of twenty successful cholecystenterostomies by means of the anastomosis button." *Chicago Medical Record* 6 (1894): 159, 232–60.

19. "Appendicitis with original report; histories and analysis of one hundred and forty-one laparotomies for that disease under personal observation." *JAMA* 22 (1894): 302, 347, 387, 423.

20. "Intestinal approximation: pathological histology of reunion and statistical analysis." *Chicago Clinical Review* 3 (1893–94): 479–558.

21. "Intestinal approximation, with especial reference to the use of the anastomosis button." *Lancet* 2 (1894): 621–25.

22. "Cholecystenterostomy." *Atti d. xi Cong Med Internaz. 1894* Roma. 4 chirurg. [etc.] (1895): 129–42.

23. "Appendicitis: further consideration of this subject, with tabulated report of cases not previously published." *Medical News* 66 (1895): 1–8.

24. "Analysis of the cases operated with Murphy button up to date." *Chicago Clinical Review* 4 (1894–95): 248–65.

25. "The surgical and medical treatment of cholelithiasis." *Medicine* 1 (1895): 139–48.

26. "Appendicitis: deductions from two hundred and seven cases operated on, with tabulated report." *JAMA* 24 (1895): 433, 482.

27. "Nephrectomy for tubercular and surgical kidneys." *JAMA* 24 (1895): 800–801.

28. "Remarks on intestinal anastomosis." *Transactions of the American Association of Obstetrics and Gynecology, 1894* 7 (1895): 384–92.

29. "Surgical clinic and demonstration [Gall tracts]." *Chicago Clinical Review* (Aug. 1895): 579–94.

30. "Surgical clinic and demonstration: End-to-end approximation."

Chicago Clinical Review 4 (1894–95): 640–44.
31. "Ovarian cyst." *Chicago Clinical Review* 5 (1895–96): 559–62.
32. "Cholelithiasis: Cholelithotomy." *Chicago Clinical Review* 5 (1895–96): 562–64.
33. "Three cases of intestinal obstruction following appendicitis." *Chicago Clinical Review* 5 (1895–96): 645–49.
34. "Report of one hundred and eleven additional cases operated upon with the anastomosis-button." *Medical News* (Nov. 16, 23, 1895).
35. "Appendicitis: deductions from two hundred and seven cases operated on, with tabulated report." *Transactions of the Chicago Pathological Society, 1894–5* 1 (1896): 87–113.
36. "Nephrectomy for tubercular and surgical kidneys." *Transactions of the Chicago Pathological Society, 1894–5* 1 (1896): 151–56.
37. "Surgery of the Gasserian ganglion with demonstration; with report of two cases." *American Medico-Surgical Bulletin* 10 (1896): 437–40.
38. "Surgery of the Gasserian ganglion with demonstration; with report of two cases." *Southwestern Medical Record* 1 (1896): 345–53.
39. "Ileus." *JAMA* 26 (1896): 15–22, 72–76.
40. "Fibromyoma complicating pregnancy: fibroma of vaginal wall." *JAMA* 26 (1896): 406–9.
41. "Intestinal obstruction from enterolith." *JAMA* 26 (1896): 432.
42. "Fibromyoma complicating pregnancy: fibroma of vaginal wall." *International Medical Magazine* 5 (1896–97): 17–22.
43. "Resection of arteries and veins injured in continuity; end to end suture—experimental and clinical research." *Railway Surgeon* 3 (1896–97): 385–404; [Discussion], 418–20.
44. "Neuro-sarcoma of the musculo-spiral nerve." *Chicago Clinic* 10 (1897): 195–99.
45. "The operative technique of appendicitis." *Chicago Medical Recorder* 13 (1897): 63–69.
46. "Vaginal hysterectomy; improved method." *Clinical Review* 7 (1897–8): 197–211.
47. "Ileus." *Deutsche Zeitschrift fuer Chirurgie* 45 (1897): 506–30.
48. "Resection of arteries and veins injured in continuity; end to end suture—experimental and clinical research." *Transactions of the American Association of Obstetrics and Gynecology* 9 (1896–97): 333–82.
49. "Resection of arteries and veins injured in continuity; end to end suture—experimental and clinical research." *Medical Record* 51 (1897): 73–88.
50. "Surgery of the bile tracts." *Southern Practitioner* 19 (1897): 481–94.
51. "Diseases of the gall-bladder." *Twentieth Century Practitioner* 9 (1897): 718–77.
52. "Ileus." *Cleveland Journal of Medicine* 3 (1898): 469–84.
53. "Choice of operation in amputations at the knee joint." *JAMA* 30 (1898): 259.
54. "Surgery of the lung." *JAMA* 31 (1898): 151–65, 208–16, 281–97, 341–56.

55. "Different phases of ileus." *Chicago Clinic* 12 (1899): 59–62.

56. "Surgery of arteries and veins injured in continuity: end-to-end suture after resection." *Comptes-Rendus du XII Congres International de Médicine, Moscou* 7(19)–14(26) August 1897 (1900): 359–86.

57. "Tuberculosis of the testicle with special consideration of its conservative treatment." *JAMA* 35 (1900): 1187–91, 1276–79, 1346–49, 1407–11, 1478–81.

58. "Resection of the rectum per vaginam." *Philadelphia Medical Journal* 7 (1901): 383–89.

59. "Fibroma of the mesentery." *Medical News* 79 (1901): 241–44.

60. "The prostate." *JAMA* 38 (1902): 743–49.

61. "Perforating ulcers of the duodenum" [coauthored with J. M. Neff]. *American Journal of Obstetrics and Diseases of Women and Children* 46 (1902): 737–64.

62. "Diagnosis of cholelithiasis." *American Journal of Surgery and Gynecology* 16 (1902–3): 138–43.

63. "Surgery of the prostate." *Illinois Medical Journal* n.s. 4 (1902–3): 810–51.

64. "Some remarks on the value of the Roentgen rays." *Plexus* 8 (1902–3): 331–39.

65. "Tuberculosis of the female genitalia and peritoneum." *American Journal of Obstetrics and Diseases of Women and Children* 48 (1903): 737–54; 49 (1903): 6.

66. "Tuberculosis of the female genitalia and peritoneum." *Transactions of American Association of Obstetrics and Gynecology, 1903* 16 (1904): 201–80.

67. "Operation for fracture of spine." *American Journal of Surgery and Gynecology* 17 (1903–4): 30–31.

68. "The Roentgen rays as a therapeutic force from a clinical standpoint, with illustrative cases." *Transactions of the American Roentgen Ray Society 1902* (1903): 84–101.

69. "Report on thirty-two cases of perineal prostatectomy: May 6th, 1901, to August 1st, 1903." *Chicago Medical Record* 25 (1903): 13, 114.

70. "Exstrophy of bladder." *Illinois Medical Journal* 5 (1903–4): 805–7.

71. "Report of a case of typhoid perforation with general peritoneal infection, and five other consecutive cases of general suppurative peritonitis; all recovered." *JAMA* 40 (1903): 977–81.

72. "Trigeminal neuralgia treated by intraneural injections of osmic acid." *JAMA* 41 (1903): 496–97.

73. "The diagnosis of gall–stones." *Medical News* 82 (1903): 825–33.

74. "On the results obtainable by operative measures in affections of the stomach." *Ann. Surg.* 38 (1903): 789–805.

75. "On the results obtainable by operative measures in affections of the stomach." *Transactions of the Philadelphia Academy of Surgery* 6 (1904): 118–33.

76. "Post-graduate work abroad: Chicago." *Lancet* 1 (1904): 47.

77. "Two thousand operations for appendicitis, with deductions from his

personal experience." *American Journal of Medical Science* 128 (1904): 187–211.

78. "Ankylosis: arthroplasty; clinical and experimental." *Transactions of the American Surgical Association* 22 (1904): 315–76.

79. "Specimen from seven months' abdominal gestation removed thirteen years later." *Ann. Surg.* 39 (1904): 464–67.

80. "A method of dispensing with rubber gloves and the adhesive rubber dam: a preliminary note." *JAMA* 42 (1904): 765.

81. "Prostatectomy: report of 51 cases operated on from May 6, 1901, to February 26, 1904." *JAMA* 42 (1904): 1408, 1557; 43 (1904): 14.

82. "Case of tetanus successfully treated by aspiration of the cerebrospinal fluid and injection of morphin-eucain and salt solution." *JAMA* 43 (1904): 460.

83. "A method of dispensing with rubber gloves and the adhesive rubber dam: second communication." *JAMA* 43 (1904): 807–8.

84. "Osmic acid injections for relief of trifacial neuralgia." *JAMA* 43 (1904): 947, 1051.

85. "Some further advances in renal surgery." *Transactions of the Southern Surgical and Gynecological Association* 1904.

86. "A case of cervical rib with symptoms resembling subclavian aneurism." *Ann. Surg.* 41 (1905): 399–406.

87. "Evolution of surgery." *Bulletin. University of Illinois* (Oct. 1905): 15–21.

88. "Ankylosis: arthroplasty; clinical and experimental." *JAMA* 44 (1905): 1573, 1671, 1749.

89. "Superior accessory thyroids." *JAMA* 45 (1905): 1854–62.

90 "Adynamic and dynamic ileus." *Ann. Surg.* 44 (1906): 141– 46.

91. "Fractures of the olecranon treated by subcutaneous exarticular wiring." *JAMA* 46 (1906): 257.

92. "Axillary and pectoral cicatrices following the removal of the breast, axillary glands, and connective tissue for maligant or other diseases." *New York Medical Journal* 83 (1906): 1–6.

93. "Fibroma of the gastrohepatic omentum in the lesser peritoneal cavity: Fibro-myxo-myoma telangiectaticum of the gastrohepatic omentum." *Surg. Gynecol. Obstet.* 1 (1905): 315–19.

94. "Technique of removal of the breast and axillary glands." *Surg. Gynecol. Obstet.* 2 (1906): 84–89.

95. "The vermiform appendix and its diseases," by Howard A. Kelly and E. Hurden; [A review of]. *Surg. Gynecol. Obstet.* 2 (1906): 245–48.

96. "The clinical significance of cervical ribs." *Surg. Gynecol. Obstet.* 3 (1906): 514–20.

97. "Indications for the technic of and results in surgery of the peripheral nerve." *Illinois Medical Journal* 12 (1907): 332–41.

98. "Surgery of the spinal cord." *JAMA* 48 (1907): 765–74, [Discussion] 826–28.

99. "Neurological surgery. A. Spinal cord; B. Peripheral nerves." *Surg.*

Gynecol. Obstet. 4 (1907): 385–500.

100. "Diffuse suppurative peritonitis: discussion." *Transactions of the American Association of Obstetrics and Gynecology, 1906* 19 (1907): 177–85.

101. "Treatment of perforative peritonitis (general, free, suppurative)," [Abstr.]. *Ann. Surg.* 47 (1908): 870–72; [Discussion], 1045–50.

102. "Tuberculosis of the patella." *Surg. Gynecol. Obstet.* 6 (1908): 262–73.

103. "Perforative peritonitis; general, free, suppurative." *Surg. Gynecol. Obstet.* 6 (1908): 575–98.

104. "Perforative peritonitis; general, free, suppurative." *Transactions of the American Surgical Association* 26 (1908): 46– 128.

105. "Perforative peritonitis; general, free, suppurative." *Old Dominion Journal of Medicine and Surgery* 7 (1908–9): 27–36.

106. "Treatment of acute diffuse suppurative peritonitis." *JAMA* 52 (1909): 988–89.

107. "Treatment of varicose ulcers by leggings." *JAMA* 52 (1909): 1033–34.

108. "Proctoclysis in the treatment of peritonitis." *JAMA* 52 (1909): 1248–50.

109. "Removal of an embolus from the common iliac artery, with re-establishment of circulation in the femoral." *JAMA* 52 (1909): 1661–63.

110. "The analysis, clinical course and present surgical treatment of tri-facial neuralgia, or tic douloureux." *Dental Review* 24 (1910): 973–82; [Discussion], 1049–63.

111. "Gallstone disease and its relation to intestinal obstruction." *Illinois Medical Journal* 18 (1910): 272–80.

112. "The arsenical treatment of syphilis." *JAMA* 55 (1910): 1113–15.

113. "The repair of injuries to peripheral nerves; with a report of two illustrative cases" [coauthored with A. B. Eustace]. *Quarterly Bulletin of Northwestern University Medical School* 12 (1910): 25–38.

114. "Fractures near and into joints." *Railway Surgical Journal* 17 (1910–11): 375–82.

115. "Organized medicine; its influence and its obligations." *JAMA* 57 (1911): 1–9.

116. "Lesions of the hip joint and their management." *Surg. Gynecol. Obstet.* 12 (1911): 200–201.

117. "The evolution of new bone and its relation to the reproduction of joints after ankylosis." *Ann. Surg.* 56 (1912): 344–47.

118. "Tuberculosis of the alimentary canal and peritoneum." *Illinois Medical Journal* 21 (1912): 287–90.

119. "X-ray findings in the differential diagnosis of early and late pregnancies," by Patrick S. O'Donnell. [Discussions, coauthored with J. B. De Lee.] *JAMA* 58 (1912): 748–50.

120. "Contribution to the surgery of bones, joints and tendons." *JAMA* 58 (1912): 985–90.

121. "Safety razor-blade scalpel." *JAMA* 59 (1912): 2127.

122. "Surgery of the bone and joints." *New York Medical Journal* 96 (1912): 1232–33.

123. "Limitations of bone regeneration and reconstruction." *Transactions of the Southern Surgical and Gynecological Association* 24 (1912): 223–36.

124. "Tuberculosis of the patella." *Illinois Medical Journal* 22 (1912): 331–36.

125. "Arthroplasty." *Ann. Surg.* 57 (1913): 593–647.

126. "Use of palate mucous membrane flaps in ankylosis of the jaw due to cicatricial formations in the cheek." *JAMA* 61 (1913): 245–47.

127. "Old ununited fracture of anatomic neck of the femur; with suggestions for the immediate treatment of this fracture." *Southern Medical Journal* 6 (1913): 387–400.

128. "Osteoplasty." *Surg. Gynecol. Obstet.* 16 (1913): 493–536.

129. "Arthroplasty for ankylosed joints." *Transactions of the American Surgical Association* 31 (1913): 67–137.

130. "Temporomandibular arthroplasty." *Ann. Surg.* 60 (1914): 127–29.

131. "Treatment of tuberculosis by pneumothorax." *Chicago Medical Record* 36 (1914): 269–83.

132. "Pneumothorax and rest treatment in the management of pulmonary tuberculosis" [coauthored with P. H. Kreuscher]. *Interstate Medical Journal* 21 (1914): 266–78.

133. "Vaccine treatment of diseases of the genito-urinary tract and their sequelae, with report of cases" [coauthored with P. H. Kreuscher]. *Interstate Medical Journal* 21 (1914): 1214–29.

134. "Arthroplasty for intra-articular bony and fibrous ankylosis of temporomandibular articulation: report of nine cases." *JAMA* 62 (1914): 1783–94.

135. "Arthroplasty for intra-articular bony and fibrous ankylosis of temporomandibular articulation: report of nine cases." *Transactions of the American Surgical Association* 32 (1914): 329–71.

136. "Myositis." *JAMA* 63 (1914): 1249–54.

137. "Fractures in the neighborhood of joints." *Journal-Lancet* 34 (1914): 231–39, 261–69, 289–300.

138. "Bone and joint disease in relation to typhoid fever." *Transactions of the American Surgical Association* 33 (1915): 645–95.

139. "Fractures." *Kentucky Medical Journal* 14 (1916): 113–34.

140. "Ankylosis of the jaw" [coauthored with P. H. Kreuscher]. *Dental Cosmos* 58 (1916): 160–86.

141. "A clinical and experimental study of the metastatic arthritides" [coauthored with P. H. Kreuscher]. *New York Medical Journal* 104 (1916): 904–5.

142. "Address of the retiring President of the Clinical Congress of Surgeons of North America." *Surg. Gynecol. Obstet.* 22 (1916): 7–10.

143. "Bone and joint disease in relation to typhoid fever." *Surg. Gynecol. Obstet.* 23 (1916): 119–43.

Surgical Clinics, Volume 1, 1912

1. "Carcinoma of the breast." 1:1.
2. "Lipoma of the shoulder." 1:14.
3. "Varicocele." 1:17.
4. "Nerve anastomosis." 1:24.
5. "Salvarsan." 1:31.
6. "Cystadenoma of the breast." 1:36.
7. "Pelvic tumor." 1:40.
8. "Exploratory laparotomy." 1:46.
9. "Fracture of the patella." 1:55.
10. "Blood-clot in the bladder; Tuberculosis of right kidney." 1:59.
11. "Charcot's disease of the hip joint." 1:64.
12. "Epithelioma of the nose." 1:77.
13. "Pelvic tumor." 1:80.
14. "Nerve anastomosis (The musculospiral nerve)." 1:91.
15. "Duodenal ulcer." 1:101.
16. "Hydrops." 1:114.
17. "Hemangioma of the leg." 1:123.
18. "Fistula in ano." 1:128.
19. "Arthritis of the wrist-joint." 1:132.
20. "Ununited fracture of the tibia (Transplantation of bone)." 1:135.
21. "Charcot's ankle-joint." 1:151.
22. "Ununited fracture of the neck of the femur." 1:165.
23. "Arthritis of the knee-joint." 1:177.
24. "Pelvic tumor." 1:181.
25. "Ununited fracture of the humerus (Transplantation of bone)." 1:193.
26. "Lengthening of the tendo achillis." 1:203.
27. "Inoperable sarcoma of the face; Salvarsan." 1:209.
28. "Cutaneous syphilis; Salvarsan." 1:211.
29. "Gastric ulcer; Secondary operation." 1:213.
30. "Ankylosis of the knee—Arthroplasty." 1:221.
31. "Volkmann's contracture." 1:231.
32. "Ankylosis of the hip—Arthroplasty." 1:243.
33. "Prolapsus recti." 1:257.
34. "Exploratory laparotomy, appendectomy, megaduodenum." 1:261.
35. "Plastic operation of the face." 1:269.
36. "Cyst in the left iliac fossa." 1:273.
37. "Trauma of cystadenoma of the breast." 1:281.
38. "Anastomosis of the external popliteal nerve." 1:285.
39. "Exhibition at Clinic of cases previously operated upon (with comments, photographs, and skiagrams)." 1:293.

40. "Impacted Colles' fracture." 1:315.
41. "Fracture of the Olecranon process." 1:325.
42. "Division of the brachial plexus." 1:339.
43. "Tuberculosis of the intestines—Laparotomy." 1:351.
44. "Cystic goiter." 1:363.
45. "Double cervical rib." 1:389.
46. "Impacted fracture of the head of the tibia with posterior luxation." 1:395.
47. "Tumor (Hypernephroma) of the kidney." 1:405.
48. "Cholelithiasis." 1:417.
49. "Typhoid spine." 1:429.
50. "Extradural hemorrhage from trauma: Excision of three and one-half inches of dura." 1:437.
51. "Pott's fracture." 1:451.
52. "Five diagnostic methods of John B. Murphy." 1:459.
53. "Acute appendicitis and pneumonia." 1:467.
54. "Chronic appendicitis." 1:473.
55. "Ankylosis of the knee; Arthroplasty; Joint infections." 1:483.
56. "Angiophlebitis of leg and thigh—Old muscular hemangioma." 1:497.
57. "Hypertrophy of the prostate." 1:509.
58. "Nephropyeloplasty." 1:515.
59. "Ankylosis of the left elbow-joint—Fracture of joint with deformity." 1:523.
60. "Tumor of the abdomen—Retroperitoneal sarcoma." 1:537.
61. "Concussion of the spine with impacted fracture of the vertebrae." 1:545.
62. "Traumatic epilepsy; Decompression." 1:547.
63. "Transplantation of bone (Osteitis fibrosa cystica)." 1:555.
64. "Carcinoma of the lip." 1:571.
65. "Carcinoma of the splenic flexure of the colon—Intestinal obstruction." 1:581.
66. "Students' clinic—Fractures." 1:591.
67. "Remarks on anesthesia made at Clinic." 1:623.
68. "Nephrolithiasis." 1:629.
69. "Cholecystitis." 1:639.
70. "Gastroduodenal ulcer—Gastro-enterostomy." 1:653.
71. "Appendiceal abscess." 1:661.
72. "Colonic adhesions simulating recurrent appendicitis." 1:665.
73. "Exophthalmic goiter." 1:673.
74. "Traumatic lesion of brain." 1:683.
75. "Trifacial neuralgia." 1:691.
76. "Tumor of spinal cord." 1:695.
77. "Chronic mastitis." 1:699.
78. "Recurrent ovarian cystosarcoma." 1:707.
79. "Retroversion of uterus." 1:713.

80. "Rectocele and perineal laceration." 1:723.
81. "Ununited fracture, Shaft of right humerus." 1:727.
82. "Osteitis fibroma cystica of right humerus." 1:741.
83. "Ankylosis of left elbow." 1:749.
84. "Ankylosis of right hip-joint." 1:761.
85. "Carcinoma of the breast (with a talk by Professor R. Bastianelli, of Rome, Italy)." 1:779.
86. "Improvements in the treatment of malignant tumors with radioactive substances (by Albert Caan, M.D.)." 1:795.
87. "Salpingitis—Pelvic Infections." 1:807.
88. "Metastatic gonorrheal arthritis of the knee." 1:825.
89. "Ankylosis of elbow—Arthroplasty." 1:833.
90. "Fracture of the patella." 1:843.
91. "Ununited fracture of femur." 1:853.
92. "Fracture of the internal semilunar cartilage." 1:861.
93. "Splitting fracture of the anterior half of the lower end of the tibia." 1:867.
94. "Ununited fracture of humerus." 1:875.
95. "Tenoplasty for obstetric palsy." 1:883.
96. "Ankylosis of the temporomaxillary joints." 1:905.
97. "Comments on cases previously operated on." 1:919.

Surgical Clinics, Volume 2, 1913

98. "Open treatment of fractures (an address and operation by Mr. W. Arbuthnott Lane, of London)." 2:1.
99. "Osteitis of femur." 2:33.
100. "Luxation of semilunar cartilage." 2:47.
101. "Floating cartilage." 2:53.
102. "Fecal fistula following appendectomy." 2:59.
103. "Medicolegal relations of physician and patient (by Dr. W. C. Woodward)." 2:69.
104. "Tuberculosis of knee: Arthrodesis (treatment of tuberculous joints)." 2:83.
105. "Paget's disease: Amputation of breast." 2:99.
106. "Acute appendicitis." 2:107.
107. "Abscess of neck." 2:119.
108. "Broad ligament abscess: Pyosalpinx." 2:123.
109. "Cerebral adhesions (Decompression)." 2:131.
110. "Fracture and luxation of the neck of the humerus." 2:137.
111. "Laminectomy." 2:149.
112. "Congenital pyloric stenosis." 2:157.
113. "Laminectomy two years after injury." 2:165.
114. "Hour-glass stomach." 2:173.
115. "Essential hemorrhage of the uterus—Hysterectomy (description of Dr. Murphy's operation for hysterectomy)." 2:181.

116. "Pyloric ulcer with hypertrophy of stomach muscle." 2:197.
117. "Duodenal block (result of adhesions following attempted perforation of ulcer)." 2:205.
118. "Active duodenal ulcer near pylorus. Bleeding about seven hours before operation—A few German statistics on the button." 2:215.
119. "Gastric ulcer, etc. A talk by Mr. Robert Milne, F.R.C.S., of London, England." 2:223.
120. "Further remarks by Mr. Robert Milne, F.R.C.S., of London, England, following an operation by Dr. Murphy for fracture of the humerus and Colles' fracture." 2:229.
121. "Contraction of intestinal anastomotic opening with extensive abdominal adhesions; Cecal fistula." 2:235.
122. "Exploratory laparotomy; Pericholecystitis; Healed duodenal ulcer." 2:243.
123. "Duodenal ulcer; Periduodenitis; Gastric ulcer with adhesions; Pericholecystitis; Gall-stones." 2:249.
124. "Exhibition of case of traumatic brachial paralysis." 2:259.
125. "Spina bifida; Meningocele." 2:265.
126. "Impacted fracture of the body of the first lumbar vertebra; Laminectomy; Rapid recovery following decompression of cord." 2:275.
127. "Ureteral calculus (Mulberry type and tunneled)." 2:287.
128. "Cerebellar tumor (marked relief following decompression)." 2:295.
129. "Osteomyelitis of tibia (transplantation of bone)." 2:305.
130. "Fracture of tibia and fibula (Lane plate)." 2:313.
131. "Periosteal sarcoma: Amputation of the leg." 2:321.
132. "Chronic trochanteric bursitis." 2:337.
133. "Later note on case of cerebral decompression." 2:344.
134. "Recurrent appendicitis—Retrocecal appendix with description of Dr. Murphy's proctoclysis." 2:345.
135. "Obturation ileus: Obstruction due to large gall-stone in ileum." 2:353.
136. "Intestinal stasis caused by band of adhesions." 2:371.
137. "Paratracheal tumor—Cystic adenoma of thyroid." 2:377.
138. "Desmoid tumor of the rectus muscle." 2:383.
139. "Plastic operation on ear (ear bitten off by a horse)." 2:389.
140. "Tenoplasty of flexor tendons of fingers." 2:393.
141. "Ankylosis of the jaw (interposition of mucous membrane flaps taken from palate and floor of mouth)." 2:405.
142. "Subcoracoid dislocation of the humerus with separation of tuberosity." 2:413.
143. "Fracture of neck of femur: Displacement of head on dorsum of ilium." 2:431.
144. "Fracture and dislocation of scaphoid and semilunar bones." 2:431.
145. "Dislocated semilunar cartilage displaced across median line of joint." 2:435.

146. "Infectious granuloma of the Caput coli—Resection of the cecum and anastomosis of the ileum to the ascending colon." 2:443.

147. "Arthroplasty of the hip—Trochanter placed in acetabulum to form a new joint." 2:449.

148. "Pott's disease (the operation of bone-grafting for its cure, as devised by Dr. F. H. Albee, of New York City). A talk by Dr. F. H. Albee, at Mercy Hospital." 2:455.

149. "Clinic at St. Luke's Hospital, Chicago, by Dr. Fred H. Albee, of New York City." 2:465.

150. "Procidentia uteri (Dr. Murphy's method of fixing the uterus)." 2:479.

151. "Cholecystitis: Symptomatic diabetes mellitus due to gall-bladder infection." 2:491.

152. "Clinic held by Dr. Murphy at Mercy Hospital for the Chicago Surgical Society, March 1, 1913." 2:501.

153. "Acute suppurative prostatitis (early drainage into urethra; Subsequent leakage through capsule, with infection of the perirectal tissues; Ischiorectal abscess; Incision, breaking down partitions between pus-pockets, and drainage; Unimpeded recovery)." 2:535.

154. "Some observations on vaccine and serum therapy from Dr. Murphy's Clinic (by Philip H. Kreuscher, M.D., of Dr. Murphy's Staff)." 2:539.

155. "The blood-supply in and around the joints (with ten skiagrams)." 2:575.

156. "Urethrorectal fistula (following perineal operation for vesical calculus)." 2:597.

157. "Laminectomy for bullet in lumbar spine—Removal of bullet (examination by Dr. Charles L. Mix)." 2:601.

158. "Fixation of knee with backward luxation of tibia." 2:611.

159. "Fracture of the femur above condyles, with non-union and overriding of the patella by the lower end of the upper fragment." 2:617.

160. "Cylindric-cell carcinoma of the breast." 2:625.

161. "Tumor of the radius." 2:631.

162. "Ankylosis of the knee-joint, with hyperextension of leg and excessive production of bone subperiosteally—Acute infections in joints; Formalin-glycerin treatment." 2:637.

163. "Postsacral dermoid." 2:647.

164. "Pseudarthrosis of shaft of humerus—Ankylosis of elbow—Wrist-drop." 2:651.

165. "Bony ankylosis of jaw, with interposition of flaps from temporal fascia." 2:659.

166. "Ununited fracture of the tibia: Removal of silver wire; Bone transplantation; Non-union of fractures—Causes." 2:665.

167. "Old ununited fracture of the tibia—Transplantation of bone." 2:675.

168. "Laminectomy for aneurysmal sarcoma (discussion of neurologic

phase of case by Dr. D'Orsay Hecht)." 2:681.

169. "Exploratory laparotomy in a case of severe ascites in a girl fifteen years of age (with remarks by Dr. Paul Chester)." 2:697.

170. "Vesical calculus with a history simulating prostatic disease." 2:705.

171. "Laminectomy for myeloma of cord (with remarks by Dr. Mix)." 2:709.

172. "Appendicitis (a talk by Dr. Norman Bridge, of Los Angeles, Cal., at the clinic, held on Wednesday, June 4, 1913) (also reprint of Dr. Murphy's article representing his teaching twenty-five years ago)." 2:717.

173. "Laminectomy for recurrent endothelioma of spinal cord—third operation." 2:733.

174. "Glioma of right cerebellar lobe—Patient kept breathing with pulmotor for thirty-four hours." 2:739.

175. "Double inguinal hernia—Some Italian statistics—Technic of the Andrews operation." 2:749.

176. "Appendicitis—Differential diagnosis; Perforations—Treatment of general suppurative peritonitis." 2:769.

177. "Osteitis fibrosa cystica of the upper end of the femur, not involving the head and neck—Transplant placed in cavity." 2:783.

178. "Cavernous angioma of the thigh." 2:807.

179. "Sarcoma of the thymus gland." 2:809.

180. "Infected bursa of olecranon; Miner's Elbow." 2:819.

181. "Healed duodenal ulcer; Constriction of pyloric zone of stomach by adhesions—Tubercular appendicitis." 2:825.

182. "Ankylosis of knee with old focus of infection in tissues outside of knee, discovered at operation—Early management of joint infections to prevent ankylosis." 2:831.

183. "Congenital idiopathic dilatation of the colon; Parry's disease; Hirschsprung's disease." 2:845.

184. "Ankylosis of hip following sore throat; Metastatic arthritis; Arthroplasty." 2:857.

185. "Calculus in the urinary bladder—Suprapubic lithotomy." 2:865.

186. "Tumor of the tongue—Tuberculoma." 2:871.

187. "Carcinoma of the tongue—Patient brought in for examination—Specimen removed for laboratory examination." 2:879.

188. "Tumor of femur; Cavity filled with Moorhof wax." 2:885.

189. "Abdominal fecal fistula following puncture of uterus by curet and drainage of retro-uterine abscess. Remarks on use of curet—Resection of Bowel—End-to-side suture—Anastomosis." 2:895.

190. "Tumor of axilla; False aneurysm of axillary artery, result of ulcerative syphilitic endarteritis, which perforated the wall of the artery." 2:907.

191. "Talk on cancer by Dr. W. L. Rodman, of Philadelphia (at the Clinic, on Thursday, June 5, 1913)." 2:915.

192. "Tuberculosis of the lung; Production of artificial pneumothorax by injection of nitrogen according to Dr. Murphy's method." 2:925.

193. "Bone cyst of the radius." 2:961.
194. "Pyonephrosis: Drainage." 2:967.
195. "Exostosis of radius and ulna." 2:979.
196. "Ununited fracture of the radius, previously plated; Transplantation of bone." 2:989.
197. "Ankylosis of elbow." 2:999.
198. "Laminectomy for tuberculoma of spinal column, with compression of spinal cord; Kyphosis and lateral curvature; Motor paralysis (neurologic findings by Dr. Charles L. Mix)." 2:1011.
199. "Subcutaneous abscess following tuberculosis of spine. Aspiration and injection of formalin and glycerin solution." 2:1027.
200. "Undescended testicle in inguinal canal." 2:1033.
201. "Cholelithiasis; Stones in common duct, with intense jaundice (talk on cholelithiasis and cholecystitis)." 2:1047.
202. "Students' clinic at opening of session this year. Illustrating Dr. Murphy's method of student instruction. With preliminary remarks." 2:1061.
203. "Students' Clinic at opening of session this year. Metastatic carcinoma of femur." 2:1065.
204. "Students' Clinic at opening of session this year. Traumatic sarcoma of femur." 2:1082.
205. "List of cases operated on and demonstrated by Dr. John B. Murphy at Mercy Hospital during the week of the Clinical Congress of Surgeons of North America (Nov. 10–15, 1913)." 2:1093.

Surgical Clinics, Volume 3, 1914

206. "Fracture of internal and external malleolus on a line with the tibio-astragaloid articulation." 3:1.
207. "Ankylosis of hip due to 'lipping' of the rim of the acetabulum; A collar of bone on the neck of the femur; Cheilotomy; Arthroplasty." 3:29.
208. "Complete bony ankylosis between tibia and patella and femur; Arthroplasty; Acute metastatic arthritis." 3:49.
209. "Tuberculosis of the testicle; Orchidectomy with implantation of paraffin substitute for testis." 3:65.
210. "Charcot ankle; Removal of articulation and nailing of astragalus to tibia." 3:85.
211. "Lord Lister and antiseptic surgery (a talk by Sir Rickman J. Godlee, President of the Royal College of Surgeons of England, at the Clinic held on Monday, November 10, 1913)." 3:91.
212. "Nitrous oxide anesthesia (a talk by Dr. George W. Crile, of Cleveland, Ohio, at the Clinic held on Friday, November 14, 1913)." 3:96.
213. "Metastatic infections (a talk by Dr. George Emerson Brewer, of New York, at the Clinic held on Friday, November 14, 1913)." 3:98.
214. "Gastric ulcer and gastric carcinoma. Gastric analyses illustrating various types of these lesions, by Mr. Herbert Paterson, F.R.C.S., of London,

England (a talk delivered at Dr. Murphy's Clinic, at Mercy Hospital, by Mr. Paterson, on Friday, November 14, 1913)." 3:101.

215. "Ununited fracture of the ulna. Transplantation of bone from tibia (exhibition of cases of bone transplantation, 130)." 3:115.

216. "Luxation of the patella and fracture of the internal semilunar cartilage; Description of Dr. Murphy's operation for luxation of the patella." 3:151.

217. "Laminectomy for traumatic compression of the spinal cord (examination by Dr. Charles Louis Mix)." 3:161.

218. "Removal of enlarged and dilated stump of gall-bladder following a previous operation, with secondary perforation of its wall by three calculi." 3:173.

219. "Radical operation for carcinoma of the breast, with description of Dr. Murphy's special technic." 3:179.

220. "Murphy's clinical talks on surgical and general diagnosis: The examination and analysis of cases." 3:191.

221. "Murphy's clinical talks on surgical and general diagnosis: Empyema." 3:194.

222. "Murphy's clinical talks on surgical and general diagnosis: Abderhalden test in tubal pregnancy." 3:206.

223. "Three cases of ectopia testis." 3:217.

224. "Cholelithiasis; Pericholecystitis; Stones in cystic duct; Cholecystectomy." 3:237.

225. "Acute pancreatic cyst (with discussion of medical phase by Dr. Charles L. Mix)." 3:247.

226. "Duodenal ulcer; Extensive adhesions; Dilated stomach; Gastroenterostomy. Description of Dr. Murphy's button operation (discussion of case by Dr. C. L. Mix)." 3:261.

227. "Goiter, a talk on the embryology, anatomy, and physiology of the thyroid." 3:285.

228. "Tuberculosis of kidney: Nephrectomy." 3:303.

229. "Vesical papillomata (a talk by Dr. Lewis Wine Bremerman at the Clinic, Nov. 29, 1913)." 3:337.

230. "Amputation neuroma with ascending neuritis; Division of right half of cauda (remarks on neurologic phase by Dr. Charles L. Mix)." 3:355.

231. "Neuroma of the ulnar nerve, Result of cicatricial compression following unrecognized fracture." 3:369.

232. "Neuroma of ulnar nerve the result of trauma incident to fracture at elbow." 3:375.

233. "Internal hemorrhoids with severe bleeding at stool, the result of a small slit in a hemorrhoidal vein (anemias: primary and secondary; Differential diagnosis by Dr. Chas. L. Mix)." 3:381.

234. "Murphy's clinical talks on surgical and general diagnosis: Talk on the importance for professional success of skill in diagnosis and prognosis. How surgery should be studied." 3:403.

235. "Murphy's clinical talks on surgical and general diagnosis: Differen-

tial diagnosis between benign and malignant breast tumors before and at operation. Varieties. Atypical forms. Clinical course. Relation of trauma to carcinoma and sarcoma. Scirrhus." 3:413.

236. "Murphy's clinical talks on surgical and general diagnosis: The differential diagnosis of gastric and duodenal ulcer by Dr. Murphy and Dr. Charles L. Mix. Value of the various diagnostic methods and their fallacies." 3:428.

237. "Murphy's clinical talks on surgical and general diagnosis: The diagnosis of pregnancy in a tube or a bicornate uterus associated with fibroid. The diagnosis of the complications and the management of the cases. Abortions. Sloughing of intra-uterine fibroid. Enucleation. Conservation of uterus." 3:445.

238. "Murphy's clinical talks on surgical and general diagnosis: The differential diagnosis of acute appendicitis, cholecystitis, and ascending urinary infection." 3:452.

239. "Murphy's clinical talks on surgical and general diagnosis: Carcinoma of the stomach at the cardiac orifice. Diagnostic talk by Dr. Charles L. Mix." 3:459.

240. "Tenoplasty; Tendon transplantation; Tendon substitution; Neuroplasty." 3:467.

241. "Tenoplasty on wrist; Adhesions of all tendons en masse; Freeing and wrapping of the superficial group in a fat and fascia flap." 3:513.

242. "Traumatic division of flexor tendons and median nerve; Tenoplasty and neuroplasty." 3:517.

243. "Bony ankylosis between ulna and humerus following fracture of olecranon; Arthroplasty." 3:523.

244. "Nailing of fracture of surgical neck of humerus after an unsuccessful attempt to secure union by bone transplantation." 3:531.

245. "Fracture-dislocation (subcoracoid) of head of humerus. Reposition of humerus head into glenoid cavity as an autoplastic graft without vascular attachments." 3:539.

246. "Compound fracture of lower third of femur, lower end of upper fragment penetrating knee-joint and resting under patella; Open apposition with lane plate." 3:545.

247. "Carcinoma of right hip, metastatic from the breast. Excision. Bone transplantation to fill the defect." 3:557.

248. "Carcinoma of right hip. Transplantation of upper third femur (same patient)." 3:562.

249. "Carcinoma of male breast." 3:569.

250. "Osteoma of the head of the fibula; Removal of tumor and bone; Transplantation." 3:575.

251. "Penetrating ulcer on the lesser curvature of the stomach; Recurrent hematemesis. Chronic pericholecystitis. Posterior gastro-enterostomy. Occlusion of pylorus by use of the ligamentum teres." 3:585.

252. "Sarcoma of the ovary with rotation of the pedicle. Differential diagnosis. Operation." 3:599.

253. "Ankylosis of the jaw. A series of pictures illustrating the steps in Dr. Murphy's operations for ankylosis of the jaw, cases of which have been reported already in the clinics." 3:611.

254. "Murphy's clinical talks on surgical and general diagnosis: Ileus, Varieties; Symptoms; Management; Illustrative cases." 3:617.

255. "Murphy's clinical talks on surgical and general diagnosis: Subserous uterine fibroid—The relations of uterine tumors to menstrual flow—Differential diagnosis." 3:653.

256. "Arthroplasty of hip (meeting of the International Surgical Congress at Mercy Hospital, Tuesday, April 21, 1914)." 3:663.

257. "Arthroplasty of hip—Partial ankylosis of the hip with bony lipping of the acetabular margin. Arthroplasty." 3:674.

258. "Arthroplasty of hip—Metastatic arthritis of the hip following tonsilitis—Lipping of the acetabulum and femoral head producing partial ankylosis—Arthroplasty." 3:681.

259. "Arthroplasty of hip—Bony ankylosis of multiple joints—Arthroplasty of the hip." 3:690.

260. "Arthroplasty of hip—Bony ankylosis of the hip, with some absorption of the head of the femur—Arthroplasty." 3:696.

261. "Ascending root neuritis following amputation of the cauda equina close to the conus." 3:705.

262. "Malignant papillomatous cyst of the breast—Differential diagnosis—Operation." 3:711.

263. "Paralytic ileus from cryptogenic peritonitis." 3:719.

264. "Old ununited Colles' fracture. Open reduction—Nailing of the fragments." 3:731.

265. "Left facial nerve paralysis of congenital origin—Macrognathia. Spinofacial nerve anastomosis." 3:745.

266. "Paralysis of the right facial nerve the result of a basal skull fracture—Fracture of the styloid process—Spinofacila nerve anastomosis." 3:751.

267. "Intra-uterine fibroid—Hysterectomy." 3:761.

268. "Paget's cancer." 3:769.

269. "Carcinoma of the rectum with ulceration—Iliac sigmoidostomy—Radical excision." 3:775.

270. "Carcinoma of the rectum with ulceration—Iliac sigmoidostomy. Second operation." 3:780.

271. "Sarcoma of humerus." 3:783.

272. "Sarcoma of humerus. Second operation. Exploration of site of the previous operation preparatory to transplantation of a piece of the tibia to the humerus." 3:799.

273. "Cerebellar tumor—Suboccipital decompression (discussion of neurologic symptoms by Dr. Charles L. Mix)." 3:805.

274. "Congenital luxation of the patella—Reduction—Excavation of a groove in the femur for its lodgement—Plastic operation and imbrication of joint capsule to hold it in its new position." 3:817.

275. "Recurrent luxation of left patella—Internal imbricating flap operation—Paralysis of right leg with a flail-joint at the ankle—Arthrodesis." 3:839.

276. "Postoperative ventral hernia following appendiceal abscess—Imbrication operation." 3:861.

277. "Murphy's clinical talks on surgical and general diagnosis: Diagnostic talk on the symptoms and signs of renal and ureteral stone, illustrated by a case." 3:871.

278. "Murphy's clinical talks on surgical and general diagnosis: The differential diagnosis of the causes of hematuria. Routes of metastasis and clinical course of malignant tumors of kidney and testis." 3:874.

279. "Murphy's clinical talks on surgical and general diagnosis: Intrathoracic sarcoma starting from the vertebral column—Differential diagnosis (examination and discussion by Dr. Charles L. Mix)." 3:883.

280. "Murphy's clinical talks on surgical and general diagnosis: A talk on the diagnosis of meningitis and the differentiation of its varieties by Dr. Charles L. Mix. Illustrated by two cases." 3:899.

281. "Murphy's clinical talks on surgical and general diagnosis: Perinephritic abscess, probably embolic in origin. Opening and drainage." 3:922.

282. "Traumatic epilepsy—Adhesions between scalp and dura through an old trephine opening—Adhesions between dura and cerebral cortex—Osteoplastic flap operation and freeing of adhesions—Subsequent coma and death." 3:931.

283. "Epithelioma of glans penis—Amputation." 3:945.

284. "Carcinoma of the corona penis with metastasis in the inguinal glands." 3:951.

285. "Fecal fistula." 3:957.

286. "Old inversion fracture of the ankle—Open reduction—Extra-articular nailing of the fragments." 3:967.

287. "Inversion fracture of the ankle treated as a Pott's fracture by an adduction dressing—Consequent adduction deformity—Operative correction and nailing of the fragments." 3:975.

288. "Old inversion fracture of the left ankle treated as a Pott's fracture. Consequent bad deformity—Open reduction and nailing." 3:987.

289. "Old Pott's fracture—Internal malleolus broken off and rotated, producing non-union—Open reduction and nailing." 3:993.

290. "Removal of nail from the right tibia and os calcis." 3:1003.

291. "A recent report from an old case of knee arthroplasty." 3:1011.

292. "Arthroplasty of the knee for bony ankylosis. Series of drawings illustrating the steps in the operation, arthroplasty of the knee for bony ankylosis, several cases of which have been reported hitherto in the clinics." 3:1019.

293. "Arthroplasty of the elbow for complete bony ankylosis between the humerus and ulna in a position of complete extension. Series of drawings illustrating the steps in the operation, arthroplasty of the elbow for complete

bony ankylosis between the humerus and ulna in a position of complete extension, cases of which have been heretofore reported in the clinics." 3:1027.

294. "Hypertrophy of the middle lobe of the prostate—Urinary retention—Prostatectomy." 3:1035.

295. "Imperforate anus." 3:1047.

296. "The use of radium and the x-rays in the treatment of cancer (a talk in the course of operating on a case of carcinoma of the breast)." 3:1057.

297. "The new offices of Dr. John B. Murphy and his staff." 3:1063.

298. "Murphy's clinical talks on surgical and general diagnosis: Fracture-dislocation of the spine at the level of the twelfth dorsal vertebra—Pressure of the lower fragment on the spinal cord—Symptoms—Diagnosis—Laminectomy—Neurologic phase by Dr. Charles L. Mix." 3:1077.

299. "Murphy's clinical talks on surgical and general diagnosis: Appendicitis in pregnancy—Appendectomy." 3:1085.

300. "Murphy's clinical talks on surgical and general diagnosis: Talk on appendicitis, apropos of a case operated on during the previous night." 3:1097.

301. "Murphy's clinical talks on surgical and general diagnosis: Recurrent cholecystitis—Cholecystotomy—Differential diagnosis of cholecystitis. Appendicitis, and pyelitis." 3:1103.

302. "Murphy's clinical talks on surgical and general diagnosis: Hodgkin's disease (by Dr. Charles L. Mix)." 3:1111.

303. "Auto-sensitized autogenous vaccines (preliminary report). By Philip H. Kreuscher, M.D., of Dr. Murphy's staff." 3:1119.

304. "Impacted fracture of external tuberosity of tibia—Chronic arthritis and great pain produced by the pressure of the intercondyloid tubercle of tibia against articular surface of femur—Arthrotomy—Excision of intercondyloid tubercle." 3:1123.

305. "Sarcoma of the right tibia—Excision—Transplantation of bone—Subsequent fracture of the transplant and development of a pseudarthrosis—Secondary transplantation of bone." 3:1133.

306. "Exostosis of interarticular surface of upper end of left tibia—Fracture of the internal semilunar cartilage." 3:1151.

307. "Multiple metastatic arthritides—Multiple ankyloses—Arthroplasty for bony ankylosis of the wrists." 3:1159.

308. "Cartilaginous exostosis of left humerus—Excision." 3:1185.

309. "Bilateral tuberculous epididymitis with abscess formation—Resection of epididymis and vas on both sides, leaving the testes." 3:1189.

310. "Gummatous tumor of the testicle." 3:1197.

311. "Perforating duodenal ulcer fixed to the anterior abdominal wall—Excision of the ulcer—Gastroduodenostomy." 3:1205.

312. "Retroperitoneal sarcoma of the upper abdomen, filling up the lesser peritoneal cavity—Exploratory laparotomy." 3:1215.

Surgical Clinics, Volume 4, 1915

313. "Murphy's clinical talks on surgical and general diagnosis: Intestinal

fistulas—A diagnostic talk followed by four cases with comments." 4:1.

314. "Murphy's clinical talks on surgical and general diagnosis: Fecal fistula following a late operation for peri-appendiceal abscesses burrowing upward behind the cecum—Excision and cure." 4:16.

315. "Murphy's clinical talks on surgical and general diagnosis: Fecal fistula following peritonitis, probably of appendiceal origin—Excision of fistula—Separation of adhesion—Resection of twelve inches of small bowel—Uneventful recovery." 4:24.

316. "Murphy's clinical talks on surgical and general diagnosis: Appendiceal concretion producing ulceration, perforation, and acute peritonitis—Gangrene of cecum—Postoperative fecal fistula—Operative relief." 4:28.

317. "Murphy's clinical talks on surgical and general diagnosis: Intestinal fistula following late operation for appendicitis; Much improvement with tuberculin injections—Operation; Recovery." 4:34.

318. "The relation of cancer research to the clinical aspects of cancer (by Harvey R. Gaylord, M.D.)." 4:39.

319. "Aneurysm of the brachial artery—Endoaneurysmorrhaphy." 4:53.

320. "Division of the brachial plexus at the level of the first rib—Suturing of the divided nerve-trunks." 4:77.

321. "Mixed round- and spindle-cell periosteal sarcoma of the right femur—Disarticulation at the hip." 4:93.

322. "Series of drawings illustrating Dr. Murphy's method of bone transplantation for non-union of the tibia, cases of which have already been reported in the clinics." 4:106.

323. "Open reduction of a posterior dislocation of the spine at the level of the second lumbar vertebra—Laminectomy." 4:109.

324. "Old compound fracture of the right malar bone resulting in loss of the external wall of the orbit—Outward dislocation of the eyeball—Unsuccessful paraffin injection—Successful bone transplantation." 4:125.

325. "Ununited birth-fracture of the clavicle—Ends freshened and united with a Lane plate after invagination." 4:133.

326. "Carbuncle of the arm—Septicemia—Metastatic pleurity—Death." 4:145.

327. "Contracting cicatrices on index-finger and thumb—Excision—Plastic operation." 4:155.

328. "Lacerated wound of thumb—Emergency case." 4:165.

329. "Malunion of a fractured femur with great angular deformity—Open reduction and plating—Hemorrhagic cyst at the fracture site." 4:169.

330. "A talk on a case of gangrenous appendicitis operated the previous evening." 4:183.

331. "Murphy's clinical talks on surgical and general diagnosis: A diagnostic talk on osteomyelitis." 4:187.

332. "Murphy's clinical talks on surgical and general diagnosis: Recurring multiple osteomyelitis and periostitis. Curettment of sinuses and granulation masses." 4:219.

333. "Murphy's clinical talks on surgical and general diagnosis: Acute

osteomyelitis of the right radius—Incision and drainage." 4:231.

334. "Bony lipping of the right acetabular margin and of the neck of the femur following a metastatic arthritis—Arthroplasty of the hip—Cheilotomy." 4:239.

335. "Carcinoma of the breast (a talk by Dr. William L. Rodman, of Philadelphia)." 4:247.

336. "Carcinoma of the colon—Diffuse miliary carcinosis of the peritoneum—Exploratory operation." 4:277.

337. "Epithelioma of the upper lip starting in an old lupus scar—Excision, plastic closure." 4:289.

338. "Intramural fibroid of the uterus—Diagnosis—Hysterectomy." 4:297.

339. "Hypertrophy of the prostate—Urinary retention and self-catheterization—Cystitis, periprostatitis, with multiple abscess and fistula formation—Perineal prostatectomy." 4:305.

340. "Spontaneous massive coagulation of cerebrospinal fluid with xanthochromia—Its significance in the diagnosis of lesions of the spinal cord and its membranes (a diagnostic talk by Dr. Charles Louis Mix)." 4:317.

341. "Spontaneous massive coagulation of cerebrospinal fluid. Comments and operation by Dr. Murphy." 4:368.

342. "Murphy's clinical talks on surgical and general diagnosis: A clinical talk on the diagnosis of injuries of the carpus." 4:383.

343. "Murphy's clinical talks on surgical and general diagnosis: Scaphoid fracture." 4:385.

344. "Murphy's clinical talks on surgical and general diagnosis: Dislocation of the semilunar." 4:394.

345. "Murphy's clinical talks on surgical and general diagnosis: Fracture of the semilunar bone." 4:412.

346. "Murphy's clinical talks on surgical and general diagnosis: Fracture of the left carpal scaphoid and dislocation of the semilunar." 4:417.

347. "Murphy's clinical talks on surgical and general diagnosis: Dislocation of the left unciform bone." 4:423.

348. "Murphy's clinical talks on surgical and general diagnosis: Transverse fracture of the left carpal scaphoid, semilunar dislocation, and fracture of the ulnar styloid." 4:427.

349. "Murphy's clinical talks on surgical and general diagnosis: Dislocation of right semilunar bone and fracture of right ulnar styloid tip—Fracture of the left ulna in its upper third." 4:431.

350. "A talk on appendicitis." 4:443.

351. "A diagnostic talk on intestinal obstruction due to a large gallstone." 4:447.

352. "Unsuccessful gastro-enterostomy for ulcer—An analysis of its causes—Suggestions for better technic (a clinical talk by Dr. William J. Mayo)." 4:457.

353. "Friction burn of left ankle—Closure of the defect by a pedicled flap of skin and fat." 4:463.

354. "A series of drawings illustrating Dr. Murphy's method of suturing a pedicled muscle flap into the laminectomy defect to protect the exposed dura and obliterate the dead space which would otherwise fill with blood clot. After intradural operations this flap transplantation diminishes the danger of infection and helps prevent the escape of cerebrospinal fluid through the wound." 4:469.

355. "Embryonic tumor of the testicle—Excision of tumor and testicle." 4:473.

356. "Tuberculosis of the left spermatic cord and epididymis." 4:491.

357. "Chronic tendovaginitis of the extensor tendon of the thumb—Excision of the tendon-sheath with the underlying periosteum—New tendon-sheath made from pedicled flaps of fat." 4:497.

358. "Painful exostosis of the os calcis." 4:505.

359. "Congenital perineal fecal fistula—Anal incompetence following operation for imperforate anus—Plastic closure of fistula and reunion of divided levator ani." 4:527.

360. "Hypernephroma of the right kidney—Nephrectomy." 4:535.

361. "Myeloid sarcoma of the left malar bone—Resection of malar with the zygoma and the outer wall of the orbit." 4:549.

362. "Malignant epulis of the mandible (giant-cell sarcoma)—Excision." 4:567.

363. "Talk of syphilis." 4:579.

364. "Tumor of the parotid salivary gland." 4:583.

365. "Plastic operation on soft parts of nose." 4:589.

366. "Plastic operation on skeleton of nose." 4:593.

367. "Carcinoma of lower lip and of submaxillary lymph-nodes—Excision of cancer-bearing area—Plastic restoration of lip." 4:599.

368. "Early carcinoma of lower lip—Radical excision." 4:605.

369. "Osteomyelitis of the maxillary antrum." 4:613.

370. "Traumatic epilepsy—Removal of hemorrhagic epidural cyst." 4:615.

371. "Extradural cerebral compression." 4:635.

372. "Ancient fracture of skull—Osteoplastic exposure—Fascia-fat transplant into dura." 4:637.

373. "Tuberculous meningitis." 4:643.

374. "Tuberculous leptomeningitis and ependymitis with necropsy." 4:647.

375. "Subacromial bursitis—Formalin-glycerin injection." 4:661.

376. "Subungual carcinoma of finger—Amputation; Metastatic carcinoma of axilla—Dissection of axilla." 4:663.

377. "Ununited fracture of humerus—Implantation;—Musculospiral paralysis from section of nerve—Neurorrhaphy." 4:667.

378. "Ancient gunshot division of musculospiral nerve—Tenoplasty—Additional note." 4:677.

379. "Ancient fracture of external condyle of humerus—Division of musculospiral nerve—Tenoplasty on hand." 4:679.

380. "Infantile palsy of lexors of hand and fingers—Tenoplasty." 4:693.

381. "Tuberculosis of sternum and rib—Excision of sinus and curettage." 4:697.

382. "Metastatic thymus tumor in breast—Amputation." 4:699.

383. "Bronchiectatic cavity—Compression of lung." 4:705.

384. "Traumatic cervical spondylitis—Cervical neuritis—Alcoholic injection of great occipital nerves." 4:713.

385. "Bony tumor of the spinal canal—Laminectomy—Spinal decompression." 4:719.

386. "Tuberculous granuloma of vertebrae involving spinal cord—Laminectomy—Interposition of muscle-flap." 4:731.

387. "Constriction of spinal cord by fibrous tissue from previous operation—Release—Duraplastic decompression." 4:741.

388. "Typhoid spondylitis in a typhoid carrier—Cholecystostomy and appendicectomy." 4:745.

389. "Cholelithiasis—Acute hemmorrhagic pancreatitis—Incision and drainage—Pancreatic cyst—Deferred marsupialization of cyst." 4:751.

390. "Fecal fistula with chronic recurrent appendicitis—Removal of appendix—Cure of fistula." 4:757.

391. "Papilloma of bladder—Suprapubic cystotomy—Resection of mucosa with cauterization." 4:761.

392. "Fracture of left patella—Open reduction and wiring." 4:767.

393. "Fracture of internal semilunar cartilage—Villous synovitis—excision of cartilage." 4:779.

394. "Compound fracture of both feet: Right foot—Fracture of astragalus and os calcis—Excision of astragalus—Osteotomy of tibia—Insertion of wedge bone-graft. Left foot—Fracture of astragalus, os calcis and scaphoid—Cuneiform resection of tarsus." 4:789.

395. "Carcinoma of gum and of submaxillary lymph-nodes—Excision of cancer-bearing area." 4:797.

396. "Carcinoma of tongue and of submaxillary lymph-nodes—Amputation of tongue and excision of cancer-bearing area." 4:803.

397. "Cicatricial contrature of neck following a burn—Resection of scar and interposition of flap of normal skin." 4:807.

398. "Recurrent luxation of humerus—Capsulorrhaphy." 4:811.

399. "Subcoracoid luxation of head and fracture of surgical neck humerus—Operative reduction maintained by plating." 4:817.

400. "Gunshot wound of arm—Cicatricial compression of ulnar nerve—Release; Division of median nerve—Neurorrhaphy." 4:823.

401. "Fracture of humerus, lower end—Fracture of ulna, olecranon process—Laceration of ulnar nerve—Operative reduction of fracture—Arthroplasty of elbow-joint." 4:833.

402. "Ununited fracture of internal condyle of humerus—Reduction of displaced fragment and retention by extra-articular drilling." 4:841.

403. "Ancient fracture-luxation of elbow-joint—Resection—Arthroplasty." 4:851.

404. "Ancient fracture of elbow-joint (olecranon process)—Resection of olecranon process." 4:863.

405. "Fracture of radius and ulna—Non-union of radius—Intramedullary and inlay transplants." 4:869.

406. "Ancient fracture of radius and ulna—Division of ulnar nerve—Neurorrhaphy." 4:877.

407. "Empyema of pleural cavity—Resection of ribs (Estlander)." 4:885.

408. "Pericholecystic and pericolonic adhesions—Release—Omentoplasty; Obliterative appendicitis and pylorospasm—Appendicectomy." 4:897.

409. "Tuberculosis of fallopian tubes—Resection; Retroversion of uterus—Correction; Suppurating dermoid cyst." 4:907.

410. "Sarcoma of ovary—Ablation." 4:915.

411. "Pyonephrosis—Incision and drainage—Subsequent nephrectomy." 4:923.

412. "Ureteral calculus—Ureterotomy—Removal of calculus." 4:931.

413. "Retroperitoneal sarcoma—Exploratory laparotomy." 4:947.

414. "Inoperable recurrent carcinoma of nasopharynx involving both superior maxillae, ethmoid, frontal and malar bones—Injection of mixed toxins—Disappearance of neoplasm under five weeks of treatment (talk given by William B. Coley)." 4:957.

415. "Metastatic arthritis of knee-joint—Vicious flexion- contracture—Tenotomy of biceps femoris with correction of deformity—Talk on autosensitized autogenous vaccines." 4:969.

416. "Ancient infection of hip-joint; Secondary flexion—Contracture of knee-joint from burrowing abscesses in thigh muscles—Operative correction—Tenoplasty." 4:979.

417. "Tuberculosis of knee-joint—Resection by the author's concavo-convex method." 4:993.

418. "Painful stumps of legs—Reamputation—Excision of neuromata—Neurorrhaphy." 4:1007.

419. "Painful stump of leg—Reamputation—Excision of neuromata—Neurorrhaphy—Thromboangiitis obliterans." 4:1013.

420. "Pott's fracture with eversion deformity: Non-union of tibial malleolus, united fracture of fibular malleolus, and posterior luxation of ankle—Operative reduction of deformity." 4:1019.

421. "Leukoplakic papilloma of buccal mucosa—Ablation of papilloma—Plastic flap restoration of mucosa." 4:1027.

422. "Recurrent leukoplakic papilloma of buccal mucosa—Ablation of papilloma—Plastic flap restoration of mucosa." 4:1033.

423. "Papilloma of lip and cheek—Excision—Plastic reconstruction." 4:1039.

424. "Congenital nasal deformity—Plastic operation—Insertion of bone-graft from tibia." 4:1045.

425. "Carcinoma of maxillary antrum—Excision of maxilla." 4:1053.

426. "Congenital (thyroglossal duct) sinus of neck—Total excision of si-

nus." 4:1059.

427. "Bilateral cervical ribs—Excision of rib on right side." 4:1067.

428. "Osteosarcoma of scapula—Total excision of scapula." 4:1073.

429. "Osteosarcoma of humerus, recurrent—Interscapulothoracic amputation." 4:1085.

430. "Cicatricial fixation of ulnar nerve in its groove sequential to ancient fracture of olecranon process—Release and transference of nerve to new side—Resection of olecranon-tip." 4:1095.

431. "Hyperflexion fracture of radius and ulna, lower third—Reduction—Bloodless fixation by extra-articular nailing." 4:1109.

432. "Extensor contracture of hands following burns—Excision of cicatricial tissue—Grafting by pedicled abdominal flap." 4:1119.

433. "Osteitis fibrosa cystica of phalanx of finger—Curettage of cyst cavity and insertion of transplant from tibia." 4:1127.

434. "Multiple angiomata—Ablation by knife." 4:1133.

435. "Biliary calculus impacted at ampulla of vater—Mobilization of duodenum—Duodenocholedochotomy—(McBurney)—Extraction of calculus." 4:1137.

436. "Adenocarcinoma of neck of uterus—Vaginal hysterectomy by Jacobson's method." 4:1145.

437. "Undescended testicle—Orchidopexy; Inguinal hernia—Herniorrhaphy (two cases)." 4:1149.

438. "Congenital luxation of both hips—Metastatic erysipelatous bilateral epiphysitis of femurs—Bloodless reduction of both luxations." 4:1159.

439. "Congenital luxation of hip—Bloodless reduction." 4:1169.

440. "Congenital luxation of both hips—Bloodless reduction." 4:1173.

441. "Old fracture—luxation of right hip-joint—Reduction after excision of head of femur." 4:1183.

442. "Coxa vara (bilateral) due to status lymphaticus hyperthymicus—Progress under conservative measures." 4:1191.

443. "I. Recent comminuted T-fracture in lower third of femur—Operative reduction—Plating." 4:1197.

444. "II. Recent fracture in lower third of femur—Operative reduction—Plating." 4:1205.

445. "Right knee: Luxation with fraying of internal semilunar cartilage and osteophyte—Arthrotomy—Excision of semilunar cartilage and of osteophyte. Left knee: Hypertrophic osteoarthritis. Talk on origin, nature, and treatment of bone and joint infections." 4:1211.

446. "Fracture of internal semilunar cartilage—Arthrotomy—Excision of cartilage." 4:1227.

447. "Foreign bodies in knee-joint—Arthrotomy—Ablation; Chronic synovitis—Resection of synovial membrane." 4:1237.

448. "Sarcoma of popliteal space—Ablation of tumor." 4:1243.

Surgical Clinics, Volume 5, 1916

449. "Congenital cyst of neck extending into axilla—Expectant treatment." 5:1.

450. "Adenocarcinoma of breast—Removal of breast with pectoral fascia—Talk on certain aspects of the metastases of cancer." 5:7.

451. "I. Ulcer of duodenum—Duodenorrhaphy—Posterior gastrojejunostomy by button method. II. Retroversion of uterus—Round ligament suspension." 5:17.

452. "Volvulus of jejunum—Untwisted; Gastric ulcer at pylorus—Posterior gastrojejunostomy by button method." 5:27.

453. "Peridiverticulitis of sigmoid—Incision and Drainage; Intestinal obstruction—Release of gut—Colostomy and enteroanastomosis by two-stage method of Mikulicz." 5:31.

454. "Urethral caruncle—Ablation." 5:45.

455. "Luxation of third lumbar vertebra with compression of cauda equina—spinal decompression." 5:49.

456. "Fracture-luxation of second lumbar vertebra with compression of cauda equina—Spinal decompression." 5:59.

457. "Tuberculosis of thoracic spine with compression of cord—Decompression of cord." 5:67.

458. "Elongation of capsule of hip-joint simulating congenital luxation—Immobilization in 'frog' position." 5:79.

459. "Ankylosis of hip-joint, dense and fibrous in type, from ancient infection—Arthroplasty by the fat-fascia flap method—Talk on technic of arthroplasty hip-joint." 5:83.

460. "Ancient tuberculosis of hip-joint—Arthroplasty—Tenotomy of adductors." 5:95.

461. "Ancient tuberculosis of hip-joint with pathologic luxation of femur—Tenotomy of adductors. Talk on origin, nature, and treatment of tuberculous vs. metastatic pyogenic joint-disease." 5:99.

462. "Ancient tuberculosis of hip-joint—Tenotomy of adductors." 5:109.

463. "Ancient metastatic bacterial synovitis of hip-joint with adduction-deformity—Three stage operation: (1) Tenotomy of adductors; (2) Tenotomy of iliopsoas; (3) Stretching by manipulation." 5:115.

464. "Osteomyelitis of femur—Sequestrectomy (two cases)." 5:119.

465. "Traumatic rupture of internal lateral ligament of knee-joint—Syndesmorraphy—Talk on certain injuries within and about the knee-joint." 5:125.

466. "External luxation of patella with a foreign body in knee-joint—Removal of foreign body—Imbrication of vastus internus aponeurosis." 5:135.

467. "Bony ankylosis of knee-joint—Three stage operation of arthro-

plasty—Talk on arthroplasty of knee-joint." 5:139.

468. "Hypertrophic villous synovitis of knee-joint—Synovial capsulectomy." 5:156.

469. "Hypertrophic villous synovitis of knee-joint—Synovial capsulectomy." 5:165.

470. "Ankylosis of knee-joint following a furuncle—Arthroplasty—Talk on the treatment of infective synovial arthritis in the acute state." 5:171.

471. "Tuberculosis of knee-joint—Resection by concavoconvex method—Subpatellar arthroplasty." 5:183.

472. "Hallux rigidus—Resection and arthroplasty; Pes planus—Elongation of peroneal tendons." 5:189.

473. "A talk on the surgery of tendons and tendon-sheaths." 5:195.

474. "Retention cyst of lip—Ablation." 5:219.

475. "Torticollis—Division of sternomastoid muscle." 5:223.

476. "Cervical rib—Excision. Collective review on surgery of cervical rib." 5:227.

477. "Hemorrhagic dural cyst—Ablation—Bibliography of injuries and diseases of the skull and meninges." 5:241.

478. "Phlegmon of spinal cord (conus medullaris)—Incision and drainage. Diagnostic discussion by Dr. Mix." 5:251.

479. "Compression fracture-luxation of thoracicolumbar spine—Decompression." 5:269.

480. "Traumatic synovitis of shoulder—Stretching of adhesions by Lorenz's method." 5:275.

481. "Disjunction of lower epiphysis of humerus—Open reduction—Fixation by nail." 5:277.

482. "Recent comminuted fracture of head of radius—Removal of head—Arthroplasty." 5:281.

483. "Recent fracture of olecranon process of ulna—Reduction and extra-articular nailing." 5:285.

484. "Musculospiral paralysis due to ancient compound fracture of humerus—Tendon-transference (flexor carpi radialis to extensors of digits)." 5:289.

485. "Tuberculous tenosynovitis of palmar synovial bursa—Injection of Calot's solution." 5:295.

486. "Ancient fracture-luxation of metacarpophalangeal joint of finger—Rectangular resection of metacarpal callus with restoration of head to position—Arthroplasty." 5:301.

487. "Post-apoplectic hemiplegic contracture—Tenotomy of hamstrings and of tendo achillis." 5:303.

488. "I. Chronic focal osteomyelitis of tibia (Brodie's abscess)—Evacuation; Contracture of tendo achillis—Tenotomy. II. Flexion-ankylosis of knee-joint—Resection by concavoconvex method." 5:309.

489. "Bowlegs (genu varum)—Cuneiform osteotomy of tibia." 5:317.

490. "Ancient traumatic loss of substance of tibialis anticus muscle—Repair by tube of fascia lata with fat—Tenotomy of tendo achillis." 5:323.

491. "Spastic (cerebral) paralysis—Tendon-transference (peroneus longus)—Elongation of flexor tendons—Fasciotomy (plantar fascia)." 5:327.

492. "Infantile paralysis (leg)—Tendon-transference." 5:333.

493. "Congenital talipes equinovarus—Tendon-elongation (Achilles)—Fasciotomy (plantar)—Tendon-transference (tibialis anticus)." 5:341.

494. "Double congenital talipes equinovarus—Operative correction." 5:345.

495. "Ancient Pott's fracture—Operative reduction—Nailing of malleoli." 5:349.

496. "Ancient bimalleolar inversion-fracture—Reduction—Nailing." 5:355.

497. "Bilateral compression-fracture of astragalus and os calcis. Right foot—Arthrodesis of astragaloscaphoid joint; Both feet—Removal of submalleolar calcanean exostosis." 5:359.

498. "Ancient fracture of astragalus—Arthrotomy of ankle-joint for resection of astragalus—Tenotomy of tendo achillis." 5:363.

499. "Perforating ulcer of heel—Excision of ulcer." 5:367.

500. "Addendum in re villous synovitis." 5:371.

501. "Talk by Dr. R. C. Coffey on certain abdominal operations." 5:373.

502. "Multiple sarcomata of skin." 5:379.

503. "Infective costal perichondritis—Resection of costal cartilages." 5:385.

504. "Diverticulum of esophagus—Conservative treatment." 5:391.

505. "Acute calculous cholecystitis—Acute pancreatitis—Cholecystostomy." 5:397.

506. "Acute cholecystitis with diffuse pancreatitis—Cholecystectomy." 5:401.

507. "Chronic cholecystitis—Pancreatic lymphangitis—Metastatic arthritis—Cholecystectomy." 5:413.

508. "Cholelithiasis, pancreatitis, appendicitis—Cholecystostomy, appendectomy." 5:423.

509. "Carcinoma of cholelithic gall-bladder—Exploratory celiotomy." 5:427.

510. "Pyloric obstruction from cicatricial band—Release; Obliterative appendicitis—Appendectomy." 5:431.

511. "Ulcer of duodenum and of jejunum—Anterior gastrojejunostomy by oblong button method." 5:435.

512. "Obturation ileus—Release by disseverance of band—Talk on intestinal obstruction." 5:439.

513. "Postoperative ventral hernia (three cases). Stone in cystic duct—Cholecystostomy (case III)." 5:445.

514. "Carcinomatosis of peritoneum—Exploratory operation." 5:457.

515. "Tuberculous peritonitis, enteritis, lymphadenitis—Exploratory celiotomy." 5:461.

516. "Fecal fistula—Closure by enterorrhaphy (two cases)." 5:465.

517. "Polyposis of sigmoid—Enterotomy—Ablation." 5:477.

518. "Perirectal sinus—Excision." 5:483.

519. "Carcinoma of rectum (two cases)—Case I—Kraske ablation; Case II—Stage I: Colostomy; Stage II: Kraske ablation." 5:489.

520. "Uterine fibroids (three cases)—Supravaginal hysterectomy, curettage (case III)." 5:497.

521. "Extra-uterine pregnancy (four cases)—Salpingectomy." 5:505.

522. "Pyosalpingitis, bilateral—Celiotomy; Drainage." 5:521.

523. "Case I—Neoplasms of both kidneys; Gastric ulcer—Exploratory celiotomy. Case II—Sarcoma of right kidney—Exploratory celiotomy." 5:527.

524. "Vesical calculus (two cases)—Suprapubic lithotomy." 5:543.

525. "Melanotic neoplasm in digastric muscle—Ablation." 5:551.

526. "Mixed tumor of parotid salivary gland—Ablation." 5:565.

527. "Bony ankylosis of temporomandibular joint—Arthroplasty (three cases). Talk on ankylosis of the mandible." 5:569.

528. "Retraction of eyeball—Fascia-fat plastic on orbital contents." 5:585.

529. "Trifacial neuralgia—Avulsion of sensory root of gasserian ganglion." 5:589.

530. "Luxation of cervical spine at atlo-axoid joint—Decompression (two cases)." 5:593.

531. "Traumatic recurrent subluxation of fourth lumbar vertebra—Albee bone-graft spinal transplant." 5:601.

532. "Tuberculosis of spine (three cases)—Cases I and II: Albee bone-graft spinal transplant; Case III: Decompression." 5:605.

533. "Fracture of humerus (anatomic neck) with loss of head—Resection and arthroplasty. Talk on technic of arthroplasty of shoulder-joint." 5:621.

534. "Fracture of humerus (condyles) and radius (head)—Resection—Arthroplasty." 5:627.

535. "Ancient T-fracture of humerus—Resection of elbow-joint—Arthroplasty." 5:635.

536. "Ancient fracture of elbow-joint with ankylosis—Resection and arthroplasty. Talk on technic of arthroplasty of elbow-joint." 5:641.

537. "Postscarlatinal arthritis of elbow—Aspiration and formalin injection." 5:649.

538. "Tuberculosis of elbow—Progress under tuberculin therapy with eventual cure." 5:651.

539. "Primary synovial tuberculosis of elbow-joint—Resection—Arthroplasty." 5:655.

540. "Cicatricial fixation of ulnar nerve from ancient cubitus valgus—Release and transference to new site." 5:661.

541. "Ancient ununited fracture of radius—Implantation of bone-graft splint." 5:671.

542. "Ancient luxation of metacarpophalangeal joint—Operative reduction." 5:675.

543. "Occult carcinoma of breast with metastases to cervical and medias-

tinal lymph-nodes, giving pressure sign—Non-operative treatment." 5:679.

544. "Sarcoma of sternum—Resection." 5:683.

545. "A series of 16 illustrations showing certain phases of gall-bladder surgery (modified from Kehr)." 5:687.

546. "Biliary calculus impacted at ampulla of vater; Contracted gall-bladder—Transduodenal choledochotomy; Cholecystotomy." 5:693.

547. "Subperitoneal streptococcic cellulitis—Talk on streptococcic infections." 5:699.

548. "Non-fusion of uterine segments of mullerian ducts—Hysteropexy of aplasic, unfused uterine strands." 5:705.

549. "Ureteral calculus—Lumbar pyelolithotomy." 5:711.

550. "Sarcoma of ilium—Exploratory laparotomy—Conservative treatment." 5:719.

551. "Ancient fracture of rim of acetabulum with displacement of head of femur—Arthrotomy of hip-joint—Reduction of fracture." 5:725.

552. "Luxation of hip-joint (two cases). Case I—Acquired obturator type—Reduction by open method. Case II—Congenital type—Reduction by open method." 5:731.

553. "Ancient bony ankylosis of hip-joint with excessive flexion-deformity—Release of ankylosis, resection of head of femur; Tenotomy of adductors." 5:737.

554. "Extensive trochanteric bursitis—Total ablation." 5:743.

555. "Bone-infections metastatic to furuncles (two cases). Case I—Pathologic fracture of femur from osteomyelitis—Reduction and dovetailing of fragments. Case II—Osteomyelitis of ilium—Treatment by autosensitized autogenous vaccine." 5:751.

556. "Traumatic intramuscular ossification (vastus internus)—Ablation of ossific tissue." 5:765.

557. "Addendum in re villous synovitis." 5:773.

558. "Talk on varicose veins and varicose leg ulcers." 5:775.

559. "Clinic for the Baltimore and Ohio Railroad surgeons." 5:799.

560. "A series of unclassified illustrations showing certain features of Dr. Murphy's operative work." 5:829.

561. "A series of sketches showing a method of treating ankylosis of the fingers by grafts of costal cartilage." 5:836.

562. "Carcinoma of mucous membrane of cheek—Ablation through Kocher incision." 5:837.

563. "Gunshot fracture of maxilla—Reduction, plating, wiring." 5:841.

564. "Osteomyelitis and malar bone—Incision and curettage." 5:843.

565. "Sarcoma of maxillary antrum—Excision of maxilla." 5:847.

566. "Osteomyelitic necrosis of mandible—Plastic reconstruction." 5:851.

567. "Cicatricial fixation of mandible following noma—Release—Interposition of mucosa flaps." 5:855.

568. "Degeneration cyst of neck (lymphadenitis)—Ablation." 5:861.

569. "Lipoma of shoulder—Ablation." 5:867.

570. "Lipoma of axilla—Ablation." 5:869.

571. "Melano-epithelioma in pigmented mole of breast with metastases to axilla—Ablation of tumor and enlarged axillary nodes." 5:875.

572. "Scirrhous carcinoma of breast—Radical ablation." 5:879.

573. "Inguinal hernia—Andrews operation." 5:887.

574. "Carcinoma of cecum—Ablation of tumor." 5:893.

575. "Chronic peritonitic obstruction of sigmoid flexure—Disseverance of bands." 5:895.

576. "Large multilocular ovarian cyst of exceptionally rapid growth—Ablation of cyst." 5:903.

577. "Lipoma of labium—Ablation." 5:907.

578. "Urethral caruncle—Albation." 5:913.

579. "Prolapse of urethral wall—Plastic resection." 5:917.

580. "Cicatricial obstruction at bladder outlet—Suprapubic cystotomy and plastic." 5:925.

581. "Hypertrophy of prostate gland—Suprapubic prostatectomy." 5:931.

582. "Tuberculosis of epididymis (bilateral)—Excision of epididymes." 5:945.

583. "Coxa vara (unilateral) due to status lymphaticus hyperthymicus—Conservative treatment." 5:955.

584. "Case I—Hyperplastic synovitis of knee-joint—Partial capsulectomy—Ablation of semilunar cartilages. Case II—Polyarthritis with rice bodies in the knee-joint—Arthrotomy with removal of rice bodies." 5:959.

585. "Varicose veins of leg—Multiple resection." 5:969.

586. "Fibroma of leg—Ablation." 5:971.

587. "Talipes equinovarus from birth palsy—Elongation of tendo Achillis—Transference of tendon of tibialis anticus muscle." 5:973.

588. "Trophic sinus of foot—Resection of metatarsal bone with excision of sinus." 5:977.

589. "Portrait of Dr. John B. Murphy." 5:985.

590. "Editor's preface." 5:985.

591. "In memoriam by Dr. E. Wyllys Andrews—Dr. J. F. Binnie—Dr. George W. Crile—Dr. John B. Deaver—Sir Rickman J. Godlee—Sir W. Arbuthnott Lane—Dr. Ernest LaPlace—Dr. Edward Martin." 5:989.

592. "The medical history and last illness of John B. Murphy (by Dr. C. L. Mix—Dr. R. H. Babcock—Dr. J. E. Keefe—Dr. W. A. Evans)." 5:1001.

593. "Osteosarcoma: Report of eight recent cases. Reference to six cases previously operated (by Albert H. Baugher, M.D.)." 5:1021.

594. "Ancient injury to skull with focal signs—Decompression." 5:1045.

595. "Harelip—Cheiloplasty." 5:1051.

596. "Angioma of lip—Ablation." 5:1053.

597. "A series of unclassified illustrations showing certain phases of Dr. Murphy's work." 5:1059.

598. "Toxic goiter with melancholia—Strumectomy." 5:1073.

599. "Exophthalmic goiter—Strumectomy. Talk on surgical pathology of thyroid gland." 5:1077.

600. "Muscular sinus of arm—Obliteration of sinus." 5:1085.

601. "Posterior luxation of elbow—Operative reduction—Extra-articular nailing—Compression neuritis of ulnar nerve—Transference." 5:1089.

602. "Ununited fracture of radius—Intramedullary transplant." 5:1097.

603. "Fracture of phalanx of finger with vicious union—Correction of deformity; Formation of new tendon-sheaths." 5:1103.

604. "Carcinoma of breast—Radical operation." 5:1107.

605. "Sinus of abdomen from gangrene of lung—Celiotomy with drainage." 5:1113.

606. "Submural abdominal abscess—Laparotomy, drainage. Talk on differential diagnosis of certain abdominal tumors." 5:1119.

607. "Fibroid of uterus—Supravaginal hysterectomy." 5:1125.

608. "Adoption of an attached pedicled flap for the cure of an impassable stricture of the urethra (by George W. Hochrein, M.D.)." 5:1129.

609. "Hydrocele—Andrews bottle operation." 5:1133.

610. "Ununited fracture of femur—Parham-Martin band." 5:1137.

611. "Osteomyelitis of femur—Amputation." 5:1141.

612. "Chronic eburnative osteitis of femur—Exploratory operation." 5:1147.

613. "Gunshot wound of knee-joint with fracture of external condyle and semilunar cartilage—Removal of bullet-fragments and of cartilage." 5:1153.

614. "Sarcoma of leg—Amputation of thigh." 5:1159.

615. "Tuberculous tenosynovitis of peroneal tendons—(1) Injections of Calot's solution; (2) Incision, excision of synovial membrane, making of new sheath from fatty tissue." 5:1165.

616. "Saline proctoclysis apparatus with a description of the apparatus as used in Dr. J. B. Murphy's clinic." 5:1169.

617. "The writings of John B. Murphy, M.D." 5:1173.

Stereoclinics

We have none of these in our collection. They apparently consisted of stereopticon illustrations for teaching.

1. "Arthroplasty for ankylosis of the knee." *Stereoclinics*. Baltimore: Howard A. Kelly, 1910.

2. "Hysterectomy for pelvic inflammatory disease." *Stereoclinics*. Baltimore: Howard A. Kelly, 1910.

3. "Technic for removal of large post-sacral teratoma." *Stereoclinics*. Baltimore: Howard A. Kelly, 1910.

4. "Treatment of Pott's fracture." *Stereoclinics*. Baltimore: Howard A Kelly, 1910.

Major Topics in Murphy's Publications

In the following list, the figures represent the number of papers or operative reports that fall into the designated categories. Many papers appear in several areas, so totals are far more than the almost eight hundred publications Murphy generated.

	Surgical Clinics	Journal Articles
Infectious Diseases	50	20
Actinomycosis	0	3
Tuberculosis	34	11
Typhoid	3	2
Tetanus	0	1
Syphilis	7	1
Vaccines	3	2
Misc.	3	0
General Surgery	220	63
Gallbladder Disease	22	12
Murphy Button	4	11
Bowel Obstruction	5	6
Peritonitis	1	8
Murphy's Drip	2	0
Appendicitis	21	12
Head and Neck	41	1
Breast	15	2
Misc.	109	7
Gynecology	31	9
Uterus	13	1
Ovary	7	1
Pelvic Infections	2	2
Misc.	9	5
Neurosurgery	73	12
Peripheral Nerves	25	10
Spinal Cord	31	2
Brain	17	0
Oncology	85	6
Orthopedics	253	30
Fractures	72	6
Ankylosis	41	10
Tumors	23	0
Misc.	117	14
Thoracic Surgery	11	1

Urology	41	11
Kidney	11	3
Prostate	5	4
Bladder	6	0
External Genitalia	17	2
Misc.	2	2
Vascular	8	8
Arteries	2	4
Cervical Rib	3	2
Varicose Veins	2	1
Embolism	0	1
Miscellaneous	37	9
Visitors	25	0
Clinics, etc.	12	0
Speeches	0	9

APPENDIX B

SELECTED REFERENCES TO JOHN B. MURPHY

Robert L. Schmitz

General Biography

1. Anonymous. *Biographies of Physicians and Surgeons,* 73–76. Chicago: J. H. Beers, 1904.

2. Anonymous. "Contributors to the science of medicine." *Medical Journal and Record* 119 (1924): 362–63.

3. Anonymous (T. S. W.). "Biographical brevities, Murphy button." *American Journal of Surgery* 10 (1930): 377.

4. Arey, L. B. *Northwestern University Medical School 1859–1979,* 515. Evanston, Ill.: Northwestern University, 1979.

5. Burgess, A. H. "Murphy, and some principles of urinary surgery." *Surg. Gynecol. Obstet.* 54 (1932): 257–73.

6. Clough, Joy, R.S.M. *In Service to Chicago: The History of Mercy Hospital,* 53. Chicago: Mercy Hospital and Medical Center, 1979.

7. Davis, L. *J. B. Murphy, Stormy Petrel of Surgery.* New York: Putnam, 1938.

8. Davis, L. "The story of a master surgeon." *Surg. Gynecol. Obstet.* 55 (1934): 398–406.

9. Fishbein, M. *A History of the American Medical Association, 1847 to 1947,* 717–20. Philadelphia: Saunders, 1947.

10. Foley, W. J. "A Bullet and a bull moose." *JAMA* 209 (1969): 2035–38.

11. Hall, D. P. "Our surgical heritage." *American Journal of Surgery* 109 (1965): 686–87.

12. Johnson, A., and D. Malone. *Dictionary of American Biography,* 353–54. New York: Scribner, 1930.

13. Johnson, J. A. "My years with Dr. John B. Murphy." *Journal-Lancet* 84 (1964): 493–96.

14. Kaufman, M., S. Galishoff, and T. L. Savitt. *Dictionary of American Medical Biography,* 547–48. Westport, Conn.: Greenwood, 1984.

15. Kelly, H. A., and W. L. Burrage. *Dictionary of American Medical Biography,* 892. New York: Appleton, 1928).

16. Lane, W. A. "The prevention of disease: a tribute to Dr. Murphy." *Surg. Gynecol. Obstet.* 42 (1926): 196–208.

17. Leonardo, R. *Lives of Master Surgeons,* 298–99. New York: Froben, 1948.

18. Magnuson, P. B. *Ring the Night Bell*, 58–84. Boston: Little, Brown, 1960.

19. Martin, F. H. *Surg. Gynecol. Obstet.* 11 (1910): 10.

20. Martin, F. H. *Fifty Years of Medicine and Surgery; An Autobiographical Sketch.* Chicago: Surgical Publishing Company of Chicago, 1934.

21. Meyer, K. A., and S. Hyman. "John B. Murphy: an inquiry into his life and scientific achievements." *Journal of the International College of Surgeons* 34 (1960): 118–26.

22. Moynihan, B. "John B. Murphy—Surgeon." *Surg. Gynecol. Obstet.* 31 (1920): 549–73. (Reprinted in *British Journal of Surgery*, Oct. 16, 1920.)

23. Musgrove, W. W. "Dr. John B. Murphy." *Manitoba Medical Association Review* 17 (1937): 201–6.

24. Nyhus, L. M., and C. Judge. "Two Irish-American surgeons: the Chicago connection." *Proceedings of the Institute of Medicine of Chicago* 42 (1989): 49–51.

25. O'Regan, S. H. *Lord of the Knife.* Amherst, Wis.: Palmer, 1986.

26. Ravitch, M. M. *A Century of Surgery,* 209. Philadelphia: Lippincott, 1981.

27. Rutkow, I. M. "A History of the *Surgical Clinics of North America.*" *Surg. Clin. North Am.* 67 (1987): 1217–39.

28. Scatliff, H. K. "Medical highlights in Chicagoland: Theodore Roosevelt and Dr. J. B. Murphy." *Chicago Medicine* 67 (1964): 397–400.

29. Turner, G. G. "Ideals and the art of surgery." *Surg. Gynecol. Obstet.* 52 (1931): 273–311.

30. Wheeler, W. C. "Pillars of surgery." *Surg. Gynecol. Obstet.* 54 (1933): 257–79.

In Memoriam

1. Andrews, E. W., J. F. Binnie, G. W. Crile, et al. "In memoriam—John Benjamin Murphy." *Clinics of John B. Murphy, M.D., at Mercy Hospital, Chicago* 5 (1916): 989–1000.

2. Anonymous. "Deaths." *JAMA* 67 (1916):629.

3. Anonymous. "John B. Murphy, M.D." *British Medical Journal* (Sept. 2, 1916): 343.

4. Anonymous. "John Benjamin Murphy, M.D." *Boston Medical and Surgical Journal* (Dec. 7, 1916): 840.

5. Anonymous. "John Benjamin Murphy." *Lancet* (Sept. 9, 1916): 485.

6. Anonymous. "John Benjamin Murphy, M.D." *New York Medical Journal* (Aug. 19, 1916): 368–69.

7. Anonymous. "John Benjamin Murphy, M.Sc., M.D., L.L.D." *Medical Record* (Aug. 19, 1916): 337.

8. Anonymous. "The death of Dr. John B. Murphy." *Modern Hospital* (n.d.): 221–23.

9. Brickner, W. M. "John B. Murphy." *American Journal of Surgery* 30 (1916): 304–5.

10. Barrett, C. W. "John Benjamin Murphy, A.M., M.D., L.L.D.,

F.A.C.S., F.R.C.S. (Eng.)." *American Journal of Obstetrics and Diseases of Women and Children* 75 (1917): 299–305.

11. Jonas, A. F. "Dr. John B. Murphy—an appreciation." *Nebraska State Medical Journal* 1 (1916): 93–95.

12. Lee, E. W. "Dr. John Benjamin Murphy." *International Journal of Surgery* (Sept. 1916): 296–98.

13. Mardill. "John B. Murphy (Chicago)." *Deutsche Zeitschrift fur chirurgie* 140 (1917): 315–17.

14. Ochsner, A. J. "John B. Murphy." *Transactions of the American Surgical Association* 36 (1918): 42–44.

15. O'Day, J. C. "Dr. John B. Murphy—a memoir." *International Journal of Medicine and Surgery* (July 1925): 255.

The Murphy Button

1. Carossini, G. "D'entero-anastomose termino-terminale." *Presse Medicale* 33 (1925): 541–43.

2. Dudley, G. S. "Use of the Murphy button in small intestinal anastomosis." *Surg. Clin. North Am.* 16 (1936): 835–38.

3. Fernicola, C. "Gastrectomia total. Esofago yeyunostomia por intususcepcion con boton de Murphy." *Boletines y trabajos. Sociedad de cirugia de Buenos Aires* 31 (1947): 931–35.

4. Forgue, E. "Les devanciers du bouton de Murphy." *Aesculape* 17 (1927): 50–55.

5. Jack, H. P. "Suprapubic drainage of the urinary bladder." *JAMA* 70 (1918): 1225.

6. Kennedy, J. W. "Resurrection of the Murphy button." *American Journal of Surgery* 5 (1928): 293–96.

7. LeVeen, H. H. "Nonsuture method for vascular anastomosis utilizing the Murphy button principle." *Archives of Surgery* 58 (1949): 504–10.

8. Lewisohn, R. "Destruction of a Murphy button retained in the stomach for seven years." *Surg. Clin. North Am.* 9 (1929): 765–68.

9. Mage, S. "Stenosis of the gastrojejunal stoma caused by retention of Murphy button." *Ann. Surg.* 104 (1936): 476–77.

10. Meyer, A. W. "Die resektion der tiefen flexur (S romanum) mit dem Murphy-knopf." *Archiv fuer Klinische Chiurgie* 171 (1932): 130–35.

11. Miscall, L., and B. B. Clark. "The Murphy button in esophago-gastrostomy." *Surgery* 14 (1943): 83–87.

12. Placeo, D. F. "Il bottone di Murphy nella chirugia abdominale." *Bollettino e memorie della Società piemontese di chirurgia* 16 (1934): 1287–95.

13. Plenk, von A. "Uber den Murphyknopf bei der abdominellen Resectio recti." *Wiener Klinische Wochenschrift* 62 (1950): 450.

14. Priton, J. B., et al. "Long-term results after portal disconnection of the esophagus using an anastomotic button for bleeding esophageal varicies." *Surg. Gynecol. Obstet.* 163 (1986): 121–25.

15. Welch, J. P. *Bowel Obstruction,* 11. Philadelphia: Saunders, 1990.

16. Wolfson, W. L., and M. J. Clurman. "A cork adjuvant to the Murphy button." *Ann. Surg.* 96 (1932): 478–80.

Vascular Anastomosis

1. Bergan, J. J., and J. S. T. Yao. *Techniques in Arterial Surgery,* 5. Philadelphia: Saunders, 1989.

2. Cuadros, C. L. "History of sleeve anastomosis." *Plastic and Reconstructive Surgery* 82 (1988): 1102–3.

3. Ravitch, M. M. *A Century of Surgery,* vol. 1, 342. Philadelphia: Lippincott, 1981.

Miscellaneous

1. Siegel, I. M. "John B. Murphy—early American orthopaedic surgeon." *International Surgery* 64 (1979): 83–85.

2. Waring, J. J. "The history of artificial pneumothorax in America: John B. Murphy makes history." *Journal of Outdoor Life* 30 (1933): 347–49, 376.

NOTES ON THE CONTRIBUTORS

All contributors to this volume are at
Mercy Hospital and Medical Center, Chicago.

William H. Blair

Senior Scientist, Department of Research

Sr. Christeta Boring, R.S.M.

Assistant Director, Quality Assurance

James J. Burden, M.D.

Senior Attending Surgeon in Urology
Associate in Urology, Northwestern University School of Medicine

Milorad M. Cupic, M.D.

Chief of Section of Anesthesia
Clinical Assistant Professor of Anesthesiology, University of Illinois College of Medicine at Chicago

Warren W. Furey, M.D.

Chief of Section of Infectious Diseases
Clinical Assistant Professor of Internal Medicine, Northwestern University School of Medicine

Michael J. Jerva, M.D.

Chief of Service of Neurosurgery
Clinical Professor of Neurosurgery, University of Illinois College of Medicine at Chicago

Gerald F. Loftus, M.D.

Chief of Section of Orthopedics
Instructor in Orthopedic Surgery, Northwestern University School of Medicine

Eugene T. McEnery, M.D.

Senior Attending Surgeon in
Urology
Associate Clinical Professor of
Surgery, Stritch School of Medi-
cine, Loyola University, Chicago

Frank J. Milloy, M.D.

Chief of Section of Thoracic
Surgery
Associate Professor of Surgery,
Rush Medical College
Clinical Associate Professor of
Surgery, University of Illinois
College of Medicine at Chicago

Timothy T. Oh, M.S.L.S.

Chief Librarian and Archivist

Alejandra Perez-Tamayo, M.D.

Assistant Attending Surgeon in
General Surgery
Clinical Assistant Professor of
Surgery, University of Illinois
College of Medicine at Chicago

Robert L. Schmitz, M.D.

Attending Surgeon Emeritus in
General Surgery
Professor Emeritus of Surgery,
University of Illinois College of
Medicine at Chicago

William A. Tito, M.D.

Senior Attending Surgeon in
General Surgery
Assistant Professor of Surgery,
University of Illinois College of
Medicine at Chicago

Michael J. Verta, M.D.

Senior Attending Surgeon in
Vascular Surgery
Clinical Assistant Professor of
Surgery, University of Illinois
College of Medicine at Chicago